CHILDLESS VOICES

Stories of Longing, Loss, Resistance and Choice

Lorna Gibb

GRANTA

Granta Publications, 12 Addison Avenue, London W11 4QR

First published in Great Britain by Granta Books 2019

A CIP catalogue record for this book is available from the British Library

9 8 7 6 5 4 3 2 1

ISBN 978 1 78378 262 8

eISBN 978 1 78378 263 5

Typeset by Avon DataSet Ltd, Bidford on Avon, B50 4JH

Printed and bound by CPI Group (UK) Ltd, Croydon, CR0 4YY

www.granta.com

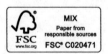

For Alan

CONTENTS

Introduction

In schoolyards and back yards around the world, we congregated, small groups of girls, pledging eternal friendship with pinpricks and promises. A handful of us wanted to focus on our careers, but by far the biggest majority wanted it all – and why not? Secure in our own bodies, by our teens we were taking or using contraceptive precautions when we experimented, lest we fall pregnant too soon and unwisely. But for a few of us, our bodies held a secret, no less life-changing than that of those girls who wore loose tops and strained to button their now too-tight jeans over fast-swelling bellies.

And so it was a long journey to this place, a curtained bed, on an NHS ward, a few minutes after retching from the effects of the anaesthetic, with my husband, solicitous beside me.

We had listened together, consummate eavesdroppers, to the girl in the bed opposite, who had told me when she arrived that she was having an abortion. She was lying in her bed, in a blue tiered gown that matched mine, chatting on her mobile phone, perhaps to a parent, saying, 'I'm just waiting for the bus now. Should be home in an hour.'

I felt sorry for her, thought it was sad she couldn't trust whoever it was with what she was going through. We spoke about her together, sympathetically, nevertheless remarking that it was odd that she was in a ward of women who were having fertility issues.

My surgeon came round to the side of my bed and stood beside my husband.

'It's not good news, I'm afraid. It's probably one of the worst cases of endometriosis I've seen in twenty odd years of surgery. The damage is extensive. There are multiple chocolate cysts and fibroids. I'm not surprised you've had so much pain. I've done my best, but I don't think it will be enough.'

In south-west India, among the village people of Karnataka, they have a different way of referring to my condition. They believe that terrible menstrual pain is caused by ghosts and spirits that inhabit the forests, and that their intervention is like 'a buffalo churning the uterus', thus preventing fertilization and causing women to be barren. I could relate to their description, because, while the words 'empty womb' mean 'without child' in many languages, during my periods my body felt more as if a creature restlessly, reluctantly inhabited it and was trying to buffet its way out. My abdomen even swelled up to accommodate its imaginary presence, without fail, for a week in every month.

Alan and I looked at each other. I think I shed tears, although I can't be sure – one of those strange tricks of memory where you can remember the exact words of a pronouncement, but not what followed, not the result.

I liked my surgeon tremendously. She was forthright and practical and I appreciated her directness. She didn't stay long, but did arrange a follow-up appointment in a matter of days, one that would be to talk, after we'd had time to speak to each other.

The girl opposite must have heard. When we pulled back the curtains, she eyed me warily. I smiled to reassure her – my own infertility was no reason to resent another woman's choice – and she gave a little wave, then said, 'I'm sorry.' I thanked her.

That 'sorry' was the first of countless expressions of sympathy that would tumble out of the mouths of friends, relatives and complete strangers in the days, weeks, years and, finally, decades to follow. With friends, with people who cared, it was comforting, but the state of childlessness was a public one that made passengers making casual conversation on trains, distant family I hadn't seen for years, new acquaintances at social events, and once even a new boss at our very first meeting, ask without hesitation, 'So, you don't have children – is it by choice?'

No, it wasn't; it isn't. But to reply and say so would herald one of two things: a well-meant but intrusive enquiry into my medical state, or, on more than one occasion, the casual, 'Did you leave it too late, then?' It's impossible to say which I grew to resent more.

If I replied 'by choice' – and I confess to having done so when I really couldn't face another dissection of my medical history – there was a whole other set of responses, some fine, some as upsetting as recounting the history of my condition. A common one, especially in the working-class area I come from, was to say, 'A career woman, then,' and to hint that I must be disappointing my parents. In other circles, where people pride themselves on their liberal attitudes and progressiveness, I'd be told, 'Well, it's not too late to change your mind, not with all the treatments available now. Sebastian – or Chloe or Portia – has brought us such joy.'

By my forties, I had armed myself with appropriate answers, bluntly challenging the appropriateness of the question. Yet through these small, petty and often well-meant, if thoughtless, exchanges, I grew to realize that, even in our progressive Western society, childlessness still carries a stigma. What I didn't appreciate was how mild that stigma is compared to the curse of being unable to have children among women, and sometimes men, in many other societies.

I travelled, and read, and shared confidences. I found childlessness was not only a historical issue, but for many people, now, in this world that we share, a real and constant dread, a shame so great that it means exile, suicide, even belief in their own damnation. I wanted to write about these people who were afraid to speak of what they saw as their own inadequacy; they were desperate to procreate, whether they actually longed for a child or not, because for them to do otherwise was to be outside of any acceptable society, to be shunned, to have no worth, to die alone. Their daily reality was beyond my comprehension, but I could at least empathize with their state.

Having children is something that defines us and perpetuates humankind. The title of parent means that you are assumed to have a publicly acknowledged responsibility and desire to care about the future. You must protect and preserve the world, for your children. Your concern is universally regarded as being beyond that of your own lifetime.

If we have loved our parents, having children is a way of ensuring that a part of them lives; if we are haunted by the idea of our own mortality, it offers comfort that this, if nothing else, is what we can leave behind, a part of ourselves.

A child can be a way of creating something with someone we love, and of making sure that the beloved's features or personality, or at least some vestige of them, will remain in the world after he or she is gone. A son or a daughter can be someone to whom you can bequeath all that you have worked for, someone to care for you in your old age, someone to bring you, in their turn, children, so that the continuity of your family seems like a surety.

In some parts of the world, having a child marks you as an adult. Without the ability to procreate, you remain a child yourself, limited in choice and freedom by the society that is threatened by your state. For many women in rural India, 'the arrival of the first child in our society symbolizes final and complete maturity of the parents as adults'.[1] Newly married women move into the house of their husband's family. The new bride is under the authority of her mother-in-law and only when she has her own children can she achieve autonomy within the household. A failure to conceive may lead to ostracism by the husband's family, which can often take the form of physical and mental abuse, resulting in what amounts to familial slavery.

But, being childless can be voluntary, a turning away from procreation for personal, religious or social reasons; some choose not to become a parent because they care about the planet and its limited, diminishing natural resources. When it is involuntary, the lack of choice can be biological or enforced by cultural or political agency. Whether childlessness is the result of a decision, a medical condition or an enforced sterilization, the treatment of the non-parent may be antiquated and dismissive, without any acknowledgement of rational or scientific explanations.

A childless person, even in what we regard as progressive societies, may still be considered selfish and shortsighted, with less of a concern for the legacy they will leave. This book looks at how childlessness is regarded from the perspective of my personal experience and the stories I encountered. By necessity, the book is genre-defying – part memoir, part cultural overview. It is a narrative about coming to terms with being an involuntarily childless woman living in Britain in the twenty-first century, but it is also, more importantly, a space for the stories of the many people whose culture and circumstances denied them a voice.

This is not a self-help book, although it may be cathartic to learn about other people in a similar situation. It could not include all of the multitudinous ways in which people experience childlessness, or even proffer a representative global sample. It presents the experiences that I listened to or read or heard about – those of the men and women who chose to share their stories. One inevitable consequence was that I became an arbiter; the choosing of which tales to tell at times meant a measuring of misery, as if I was adding to the abnegation, the discarding of a tale, by selecting one and not another.

This book hopes to raise awareness, to educate and to make connections across cultures and countries and continents. Stories that have been neglected or silenced will be told and someone who has been forgotten or disregarded or discarded may gain just a little more importance in our collective understanding of the world. It is also my experience, or at least part of it. For a time, I was mindful of a line from Beckett's *Footfalls*: 'There is no sleep so deep I will not find you there.'[2] My unborn child, the one who will never be, finds me even in sleep. But it was a brief yearning of a few years for me; time passed and there was no more longing, just a sense of absence. But it isn't like that for everyone.

The structure of the book reflects the reasons for childlessness and globally idiosyncratic attitudes and perceptions but also looks for commonality between consequences and experience. It begins with 'Those Who Long', which explores my own experience in the Middle East, where a small group of women I encountered afforded me a glimpse of how cultural particularities change the childless experience. Books and articles on the subjects of infertility and polygyny, even a plethora of statistics and factual documentation, did not prepare me for their stories. But these were only some of the women who long for children. There are cultures where the need for a child is so great that a life without one is unimaginable. To be without children is to be without status or respect; the women long not only for a baby but for a place in society.

In the quest for a child, men and women usually start out with faith that it will eventually be possible, that setbacks are only temporary. This hope can see them turning to religion or spirituality, science or doctors, for an answer, but in both cases the hopeful may be exploited. Childless men and women have for centuries looked to talismans and shrines to bring them offspring. In 'Those Who Believe' I look at some of these practices, both historic and current; there are harmless good-luck charms redolent of the wish for land that is fertile, but there are also terrifying practices that are a travesty of ancient mystical beliefs. From birds denied flight to the breast milk of a virginal mother, they represent the myriad forms of hopefulness and punishment, belief and exclusion.

Within my own culture, I look at the hope that is offered by modern science, the fertility treatments that are rejected by those with some religious beliefs but are embraced by others, and I consider the inequality in the availability of such treatments – in Britain the 'postcode lottery' and, in the USA, an online competition to find the person, or couple, most deserving of free treatment. Through it all is the dismaying fact that there is limited access to free treatment for a condition that many even refuse to see as a medical problem.

Other people may have been fortunate in their biology but less lucky in the country of their birth. Compulsory sterilization has been common practice in Eastern Europe among the Roma population for decades, as a way to curb the Roma cultural tendency to favour large families. Similarly, the practice of female genital mutilation has rendered some young women incapable of giving birth. The chapter 'Those Who Were Denied' looks at people who have been made infertile by political or cultural acts; we observe how the chance to have children – this most personal of issues and life decisions – may be controlled by others.

Despite the implacable consequences in some societies, we will learn that there are a few who manage to adapt. Sometimes a whole culture changes as a result of awareness, education or political change; at others an individual finds a path for himself or herself. These stories of resistance and agency offer real hope.

There are also the childless parents, whose child or children have died. Bereavement after illness or after a violent act leaves mothers and fathers who must navigate the world both as the parents they will always be and as the childless families they have become. Parents of missing children feel their roles suspended, tantalized by the possibility of their child's return. In the Aboriginal communities of Australia, children are still taken from their families and communities by the state. The parents left behind grieve, but are also angry and defiant; the theft of a child is felt not only as a suspension of the parenting role, but as a culture interrupted, closer to being lost altogether.

'Those Who Choose' considers the child-free, those who have made a decision not to have children. Lifestyle choices, environmental concerns or lack of interest can all lead people to choose to be childless. Some religions honour celibate men or women who choose childlessness as part of the religious vocation. An interview with a Christian nun shows how this can lead to a greater respect and a higher position in society, in contrast to many of the other childless groups in the book. Yet the faiths of these very devout individuals may in other circumstances openly condemn others who choose childlessness. In 2015 Pope Francis addressed crowds in St Peter's Square in Rome, saying, 'The choice to not have children is selfish. Life rejuvenates and acquires energy when it multiplies: it is enriched, not impoverished.' He warned that, in the end, a childless marriage 'comes to old age in solitude, with the bitterness of loneliness'. Yes, studies have looked at the ageing childless population in the West and considered some of the difficulties, even confirmed the unhappy correlation of old age and loneliness, but having children is in no way a guarantee of company in later years, nor should any individual, community or religious organization expect it to be.

I explore how everyday discrimination against the childless may be casual and unthinking but at other times is legislative and more sinister. Thus, care for those who are elderly is a social issue too often assumed to be the responsibility of offspring, while legislation on matters such as tax and inheritance may openly disfavour those who are childless.

In my travels, I found solidarity with others who share my own involuntary condition. I encountered initial wariness from some of those who had made the choice to be without children and thought I might somehow resent it, and I experienced true sorrow when listening to those who had become childless when their nation decided that other people were somehow better able to raise their children. I met with hostility in societies where my childlessness branded me as threatening or as cursed as the women I had come to speak to, and I was thwarted in supposedly progressive countries where my interest in their murky past was seen as a preoccupation with something best forgotten. I held hands with women and wept with them; I looked at faded photographs across a wavering Skype connection and tried really to see the people as they are and as they had once been. Above all, I tried very hard not to speak for people but to listen to them and let others hear their voice.

My emotional journey begins and ends in the home that I share with my husband, but it takes in five continents, countless conversations, shared confidences and quiet reflections. It is not always a happy expedition, but in certain moments there is something akin to joy, when shared experience overcomes all limitations of culture, language, even history, and I found that people would turn to me to tell their stories. Because of the attitude of their societies, these people had come to feel as if their existence was pointless, an aberration. They had felt that being childless denuded them of any identity, because the only one that mattered and had value, was that of mother or father. They had not imagined that anyone might want to learn about them, listen to them. I know that they were mistaken.

1

Those Who Long

The journey towards acceptance of our childlessness, the metaphorical act of travelling, began with a flight and a physical relocation that saw my husband and me leave our country to take up temporary lives in Doha, Qatar, where I'd been offered a place to teach at the university. We travelled with a rescue Bengal cat, Ivanhoe, our gift to ourselves that was the embodiment of so much pop psychology, lots of luggage, and a trunk of manuscript papers because I was working on an idea for a new book.

I was not a stranger to the Middle East, having spent some time in Lebanon while researching a biography of Lady Hester Stanhope. But I was well aware that the chaotic pluralism of Lebanon, which I loved, would be a marked contrast to the Muslim State of Qatar. There were similarities, however; like Beirut and Sidon and Tripoli, although for altogether different reasons, Doha had building work going on everywhere. Even our compound was not quite complete when we arrived and we were put up in temporary accommodation in a flat close to the airport with a view of a waste ground, a soon-to-be building site, where yellow emaciated wild dogs scavenged for food and water and howled into the small hours of the morning. But whereas the Lebanese cities were rising, phoenix-like, from the ravages of civil war and bombings, Qatar was growing to display its wealth, funded by its gas reserves, constructing ornate, ever higher buildings, like a peacock opening its tail.

Naively, in retrospect, I had thought of Doha as a modern, Westernized city and had not expected the niqab to be quite so all-pervasive. But it was. In those first days, I felt that the black abaya, the full-length shapeless dress, and the niqab, covering the whole head and face apart from a narrow eye slit, would prevent me ever knowing any women at all. But it became familiar soon enough and I learned to read the slight scrunching of the eyes which meant a smile, the widening for surprise, the dark dullness of sorrow and sympathy. Unlike the black abayas I had seen Muslim women wear in London, in Qatar they were ornately decorated at the edges of the sleeves, on the back or down the seams. Fashions for these decorations came and went. While I was there a Japanese theme was popular and, for a time, kimono-shaped sleeves adorned the Arab dress, with ornate embroidery reminiscent of a Hiroshige landscape.

I started wearing an abaya to work on my second week. It was a practical decision at first. Western-style clothes were too hot, too tight and made men stare at me in the malls and communal spaces of the university. Under my abaya, loose and flowing, I wore only underwear, and I relished the coolness and anonymity it afforded me. But while it magically rendered me invisible to disapproving or curious eyes, my transformation had a different effect on the women at work, my students and their families. As if by some tacit agreement, the abaya, and the message that the Qatari took from it – that I was trying to embrace the new culture – encouraged people to speak to me, to befriend me. Women who passed in the street would openly comment that it was lovely to see a Westerner wearing traditional dress. My students admired my choice of abaya – my first one was edged with white crystalline stones that caught the sun when I moved – and their parents invited me for tea.

I was grateful for the kindness but those invitations meant I had to face the social challenge of being childless in a society where a woman is defined by her role within the family. Despite its carefully promoted media image as a country of modernity and change, Qatar, like Kuwait, the Arab Emirates, Bahrain, northern Yemen and Sudan, has a traditional (*al-taqlidiyyya*) constitution, which ties a woman's identity to her position as a mother; in each of these countries her protection by the law is explicitly guaranteed by her fulfilment of that role.[1] Thus Article 21 of the 1972 Qatari constitution states: 'The family is the basis of the society. A Qatari family is founded on religion, ethics and patriotism. The law shall regulate adequate means to protect the family, support its structure, strengthen its ties, and protect maternity, childhood, and old age.'

In such a society, the experience of childbirth is a fundamental commonality that is impossible to avoid in conversation, and not just in informal social settings. For example, two female academics meeting in a formal situation for the first time would discuss how many children, of what gender, they each had, in a way that women in the West might be reluctant to do with relative strangers in a working environment. I was still getting used to the diagnosis of infertility, but I was determined not to let it get in the way of daily interaction, so I cultivated a polite expression of sadness when asked about my own children, my own births. I was content to listen to other women's accounts of their maternity experience and less willing to speak about what I still saw as my own failing. I made it clear from my demeanour that it was not by choice, but from necessity, and found that the gentle enquiries melted away, like snow under the desert heat, in the intimacy of the tea houses in the old market place where I often met my new friends and acquaintances in the early evening.

So it was for a time, until I met Fatima's mother, or rather one of her mothers.

Those Who Long: Sharing

Fatima was one of my students. Her mother, Halima, came to collect her after class and she invited me to have coffee. Because the cafe where we sat was in the women's section of the university, Halima unfastened her niqab veil, and I saw a generous smiling mouth with gapped front teeth that made her seem younger than I knew her to be. I told her that her daughter was doing well, was a lovely member of my seminar group. When we'd finished our cake, she said, 'She's not my daughter, you know.' I apologised, said I'd misunderstood. But she interrupted – no, I hadn't. She was married to Fatima's father, was his first wife, but was barren (she used precisely that word, a word I detest), and so when he took a second wife, Ayesha, their child became a shared daughter.

They lived together – Mohammed, his two wives and the much-loved Fatima. Halima pre-empted my response, said she had been to London, and that she knew I must find the idea of plural wives a difficult one. I nodded, and said, encouragingly, 'But it works for you? In your culture, I mean?' 'No,' she said, 'but it's better than the alternative. I still have a husband, a home, a child. I don't mind the other wife, although we're not friends, and, of course, I cried for days without stopping when my husband told me he was going to marry again. But he's a kind man; he didn't divorce me. That would have been much worse. My family are old-fashioned, they'd have thought it was a punishment from Allah. God knows where I would have ended up.'

Polygyny is sanctioned by Islam but is rarer in Qatar than in many other countries of the Middle East. In 2010 a newspaper article in *Al Arabiya News* reported that the number of new polygynous marriages in Qatar had dropped to just 4 per cent.[2] Various contradictory causes were suggested: the increasing economic independence of women versus a decrease in personal wealth which made providing for more than one wife difficult financially. One researcher, Ibrahim Gomaa, was displeased by the change: 'The Qatari society did not suffer the problem of spinsterhood before. Now this problem will be magnified as polygamy drops, especially that the Qatari society is small and conservative.'

Sex outside of marriage, and thus procreation, is illegal in Qatar, and punishable by sentences ranging from the death penalty to lashes and imprisonment. One 'problem' of spinsterhood is that unmarried Qatari women are thus denied, by law, a sex life as well as the possibility of assuming the culturally defining roles of wife and mother.

Islamic law expressly sanctions taking another wife in order to beget children, and there is a Hadith, a saying of the Prophet, in which Mohammed instructs a man who comes to him three times that he should not marry a childless woman, advising him to 'marry the one who is loving and fertile'.[3] I heard several stories, from my students, from Halima and her friends, of infertile first wives who actually asked their husband to take another spouse, but I never actually met anyone in that position.

The medical definition of infertility is simply the inability to conceive after twelve months of unprotected sex;[4] it is therefore a temporary state, one that offers every hope of resolution. Yet the commonly understood definition denotes a permanent condition. Many people use 'infertile' as a kinder alternative to words such as 'sterile' or 'barren'. To me, when Halima called herself barren, it sounded as if she was flaying herself for her own failure. Months later, when I knew her better, I asked her outright. I wondered if it was a question of language (although her English was excellent) and if the sense of words like 'barren' had become conflated with 'infertility'? But she said, '*La*,' and nodded, which in Arabic culture means no, and then lifted the red sequin-embellished arm of her abaya, gesturing at the dusty ground around the university. 'I am like that,' she said, 'the barren place where nothing grows. Ayesha is like the palm trees at our reception. See how the green parakeets congregate and sing and nest in her branches.'

The living arrangements in polygynous households are markedly different. In some cases, the two wives live in distant houses, barely aware of each other, knowing only that when their husband is absent, he is with the other wife. In wealthier families, the wives can have separate households within the same large compound, shared with their husband's family. Halima's family shared a detached two-storey building, set just off the new highway on the outskirts of Doha. It was new, not more than twenty years old, and they had moved there when it was first built, shortly after Ayesha gave birth to Fatima. The downstairs consisted of a large open living and dining space, where I was entertained, with a small kitchen and maid's quarters through an arched wooden door carved with passages from the Koran. Upstairs there was a bathroom and four bedrooms: one for Fatima, one for each of the wives, and a large master bedroom for Mohammed when he wished to be alone. Halima once told me, shyly, giggling, that when she and Ayesha first lived together, they would compete not for visits from their husband but for invitations to the splendour of this room.

As a guest in their home, I was struck by the apparent ease of their arrangement. There was no obvious tension between Halima and Ayesha and, even more surprisingly, Fatima did not seem to be closer to either her birth mother or her stepmother. Mohammed appeared only briefly, when we were being served dates with that lovely hot, spicy drink that Qataris call Arabic coffee, which is made of cardamom seeds. He told me proudly that Ayesha had grown the dates herself in their other Egyptian home. He was perhaps unaware of the irony, but I looked at the fat, sweet, sticky brown fruit, and saw, as with the palm trees, another metaphor for the multitudinous meanings of fertility.

Through Halima, I met other women with similar arrangements and asked them to share their stories. Their religion and culture presented polygyny as a solution to the societal difficulties caused by childlessness, but too often this brought other, equally challenging problems for the women.

In the wider region, just as in Qatar, there was a varied understanding of the state. A Kuwaiti study showed that better-educated couples cite health, marital, psychosexual and nutritional factors as causes for their childlessness, but among illiterate and itinerant participants, infertility was a curse of God or the result of evil spirits, witchcraft, curses and the supernatural.[5] Unsurprisingly the attitude of Kuwaiti society towards those affected was also polarized by socio-demographics. In Saudi Arabia, infertility is a social problem as well as a medical one. A study published in the *International Journal of Medicine* details the kind of experience that women often face: 'Women are verbally or physically abused in their own homes, deprived of their inheritance, sent back to their parents, or even have their marriage dissolved or terminated if they are unable to conceive.'[6] Of the participants interviewed by the researchers, 85 per cent attributed their infertility to black magic with a further 80.7 per cent blaming djinns and other supernatural causes.[7]

Halima was a devout Muslim and attributed her own childlessness to the will of Allah. One of the first phrases I learned in Arabic was *inshallah*: 'God willing' or 'according to the will of Allah'. The phrase was used by everyone, but to me it seemed the infertile women used it most of all, littering their conversations with the phrase as a mantra both for where they were, and for what might be possible if God so allowed. As the *surah* says: 'He bestows female (offspring) upon whom He wills, and bestows male (offspring) upon whom He wills. Or He bestows both males and females, and He renders barren whom He wills. Verily, He is the All-Knower and is Able to do all things.[8]

Two of the women that Halima introduced me to, within just a week or so of our first meeting, were Leyla and Noor, both first wives. In Leyla's case, she had always expected her husband to take more than one wife because she had been raised in a polygynous family. She extolled the comfort that she found in sharing a house with the second wife's children; she thought it callous that such an arrangement was impossible in the West.

But for Noor, the presence of the second spouse was a constant, painful reminder of her own inadequacy. She spoke often of a jealousy that at times swelled up inside her and made her feel she could not breathe. She thought of both the resentment and her inability to have a child as punishments for some unknown and thus unacknowledged sin. She said on more than one occasion that if she could only find out what harm she had done, and make amends to Allah, then perhaps a baby would begin to grow inside her. In Noor's home, a concrete house with arching mosque-like windows on a family compound where dusty wide roads were broken up by beds of struggling desert plants, the two wives circled each other, wary as cats, and I thought it a hellish, *huis clos* way to live. Noor's prayers were punctuated with *dua*, special requests that she might bear a child, and, despite the fact that she was now fifty and past the menopause, she clung to the hope of a miracle, a gift from God.

In common with many of her countrywomen, in an irony she could not see, Noor guarded the chastity of her servants with threats of lashes, constantly fearful that they might 'breed' (she used that exact word) with each other in the illicit, illegal act of unmarried sex. The threats were not unusual. In the region, Asian or Filipina girls who become pregnant when in service are asked to produce their marriage certificate. If they cannot, they face lashes then deportation.[9]

We met on occasion, Noor, Leyla and I, away from the

university, in Doha's Souq Waqif. In the mid 2000s, much of it was a ramshackle place, thick with the smell from the open barrels of the spice sellers, with stalls selling woven rugs, Arabic dress, camel souvenirs and shisha tobacco. Other stalls were presided over by hooded falcons, who scrutinized customers through the slits in their head coverings, as if they might buy you instead of the other way around. I often shopped at the souk for *oud*, the tree bark that is burned in homes all over the Middle East to fill them with heady sweet perfume.

One of the tea houses we favoured was run by an Iranian man. He served finely layered pastries, thick with honey and almonds, delicious with mint tea, in a space bedecked with artefacts relating to the history of pearl fishing in Qatar – the side of a dhow, the leather sheath that protected a diver's hands or feet from rocks, some empty shells.

I arrived a little late one November evening, having been delayed by sudden heavy rain – that rarest of events in Doha – which had reduced the traffic to a crawl. I immediately saw someone I didn't recognize chatting with Noor and Leyla. Her name was Khadiga. Her abaya, unlike those of my friends, was without adornment; her head was covered in the close fashion so that the scarf was tight around her face rather than pulled back behind her neck; and, unlike all the other women I knew well, even the eye slit of her niqab was veiled with black chiffon. She smiled when I arrived and greeted me in perfect American-accented English: 'I have heard so much about you – your interest in us, the childless women. I'm Khadiga. It's lovely to meet you at last.'

Khadiga was not anyone's wife. It was the first thing she told me about herself. She was a successful banker and lived

near the new Villaggio shopping centre with her sister, two
nephews and her brother-in-law. 'Halima tells me you write
books.' I nodded somewhat bashfully. 'So you need to know
about the evil eye.'

Ayn talismans – blue or green eye-shaped pendants with
black pupils, thought to ward off ill-wishing and bad luck –
were sold everywhere, from upmarket shops to ramshackle
stalls in the souk, depending on their intricacy or materials.
Belief in the *ayn* is well established in Islam, with Arabic
scholars commenting that Mohammed said, 'The evil eye is a
reality.'[10] When a compliment was paid, even in English, the
remark was usually followed by the Arabic phrase *mashallah*,
'God has willed it', a way of protecting against the evil eye
of envy.

Khadiga explained that the envy of a childless woman –
her longing to have children – was seen by many as something that could bring harm. The eyes of the childless
woman were malicious, threatening to bring sickness to an
infant, misfortune to a son, shame to a daughter. The veil
that covered Khadiga's eyes took on a darker significance in
my mind. It might just symbolize her wish not to be looked
upon lest she stir men's desires, or, as many students had told
me, it could create a calm place removed from the turmoil of
a world that was at times difficult to navigate. Nevertheless,
I pictured it now as some outward reassurance of Khadiga's
harmlessness, a way she could show the childbearing that
she meant them no harm: a device for diminishing the
power she had, unwittingly, unwillingly, in their imagination.

Khadiga's story sounded like something from another,
more ancient time. Her whole family had moved from the
countryside to the city because their original house was close

to a school and if she was seen there by waiting parents, they would call names and hiss at her. 'It probably wouldn't happen in Doha,' she said, almost defensively. 'And I'm so fortunate that my sister and her husband came to the city, in part so that I could be free of this. I can't really complain. Think how much more difficult it would be if I was alone.'

Khadiga had had a complete hysterectomy in her early teens. I never asked for details of the medical condition that necessitated it. I was at that time still chary of discussing my own health history and assumed that many other women might feel the same. But she believed that she could not marry anyone knowing that she was unable to carry a child. 'And in any case,' she said, sipping her mint tea, carefully lifting the cup beneath her veil, 'who would want a barren woman?'

Yet she did have a sense of her own value. She loved her work, was proud of what she had achieved and clearly adored her nephews. Women in Qatar, unlike in neighbouring Saudi Arabia, were active in the workplace, could drive cars, and this modernity brought a sense of life worth living, even if it was not a life that any of them would have chosen.

Those Who Long: Dying for a Baby

The stories in this book are the result of interlinked searches, fragile chains of connections and information. At times, these pathways of happenstance and serendipity seemed so unlikely that I was left with wonder that I had ever found them. And yet it is such random chance encounters that make our lives. I met my husband in a bar near Kings

Cross, London, a place where neither of us had ever been, just because a member of each of our separate groups of friends had wanted to stop there to use the toilets. More than eighteen years later, we are still together, but I wonder what might have happened had it not been for that chance encounter. I would still be childless – that was decreed by my biology – but would I have found such acceptance and kindness from anyone else?

Without emotional support the consequences of child-lessness can be even more devastating. In developing countries there is compelling evidence of an association between female suicidal behaviour and childlessness.[11] Dr Sayeed Unisa, from the International Institute for Population Sciences in Mumbai, observes: 'There are more negative, social, cultural and emotional repercussions for childless women [in India] than for any other non-life-threatening condition.[12] These include physical violence from their husbands, the threat of divorce, comments and abuse from their community, forcing them to become 'social recluses in many cases' and leaving them isolated and ashamed.[13]

Research from the Maharaja Sayajirao University of Baroda in India concurs: 'When a woman is unable to conceive, she is stigmatized and rebuked by family and society . . . society inflicts multiple psychological tortures by labelling them "incomplete" or "worthless". A childless woman is predisposed to being deserted or divorced. The incidence of physical violence experienced by childless women is high.'[14]

Statistics show that, in India, pregnancy and motherhood offer some protection against suicide – rates are significantly lower than they are for childless women.[15] Indian newspapers such as *The Times of India*, *The Hindu* and Calcutta's *The Telegraph* report on the prevalence of suicide, giving the personal stories of the many women, and in one case both a man and a woman, who have lost the wish to live because they could not create new life.

In New Delhi, a woman of just twenty-eight, depressed by her inability to conceive, jumped from her second-floor home. Another headline: 'Childless Woman Sets Self on Fire, Dies'. Sampa was thirty, had been married for four years to Bapi, a salesman, but, despite their hopes, their longing, they remained without any children. In Sonaltand Village, Kandra, in the north-eastern Indian state of Jharkhand, a middle-aged man called Jitvahan went to take his morning bath, only to find Lalita, his wife of ten years, hanging from a noose made of nylon rope. He screamed and the neighbours came. It was 7 a.m. and they were in various state of awakening, or preparedness for the day. Together they took Lalita down and carried her lifeless body to the home of a nearby medic, but it was too late. They were not as poor as many others in their village; Jitvahan had a grocery shop which did well, so his wife had tried infertility treatment in three different towns. But it had been to no avail. 'She told me she did not want to live if she could not have children,' he said.

Basavaraj and Sudha Karigar were married for eight years. After the first year, they began looking for medical help to conceive – from hospitals, doctors and, later, from Hindu priests, who told them to offer 'puja', or prayer rituals, to 'powerful' deities. Puja can be used to mark an auspicious event, like the birth of a child, but also to revere a god so he or she may bestow something much longed for on you. But for Basavaraj, hope seemed to have got lost amidst the devotions and the medical interventions, and so, one night, while his wife was asleep, he hanged himself. Sudha found him and ran to the home of her relatives, who rushed to remove Basavaraj's body. Sudha remained at home. All alone, she doused herself with kerosene and set herself alight. She was dead before they returned to her.[16]

The news stories are tantalizingly vague. The domestic circumstances, the lives leading to despair of the falling, burning, hanging women who killed themselves, seemed unknowable. For Sampa, were there miscarriages, I wondered – hope offered then snatched away – or simply an unbroken sequence of monthly bleedings leading to her suicide? Did she know if there was something wrong, or assume that there had to be; had she had tests; had her husband? I imagined their first year of togetherness, the love-making that they assumed would bring a child, perhaps a sad turning to frantic coupling as the years passed, half-hopeful, half-enjoyed.

Then, through the most tenuous connection with India, a woman wrote to me. It was the most unlikely of links – a passing mention from someone I had once worked with to a relative, to a friend of their cousin.

Bhakti was accompanied by her son on Skype.[17] I can't speak Hindi so he had offered to translate for us. A tiny Indian lady in a cream sari, accompanied by a moustached man in an immaculate suit, appeared on my screen. Ravi spoke perfectly enunciated English and began the introduction by making a slight bow. I insisted he didn't call me Dr Gibb, and then regretted it, because he immediately looked uncomfortable with the informality of using my first name.

Bhakti began her story in a rush of sounds, incomprehensible to me, but I could see the emotion on her face, carefully held in check, behind a dam of polite communication and formality. Her daughter Sur made a love match with a boy she had known since childhood. Lakshman was two years older, from a neighbouring village, and, with the approval of both sets of parents, they married when Sur was twenty-one. 'We liked her husband's family,' Ravi translated for me. 'They were good people and close by, so when Sur moved in to live with them we were happy, because we knew that we might still see her from time to time. At first they were good in-laws too. Yes, it was a traditional house, but Sur told us she was happy that she shared the work with Lakshman's mother and didn't suffer in the way that some of her contemporaries did – girls who became little more than servants in the family home of their husbands.'

Bhakti's face crumpled a little, her voice wavered, and Ravi, solicitous, turned to her and placed his hand on her arm. I was touched by his care and gave a sympathetic half-smile. Bhakti smiled back – a beaming grin that seemed at odds with all the emotion I had heard. She spoke to Ravi and he too smiled. 'She says she is happy that you want to know her story. It's been a few years since Sur died but we don't want to forget her. Perhaps your book will make people think about her for a few minutes.' He paused. Mother and son exchanged some words. 'Sorry, I was just saying to her that what she said wouldn't help with your story, but she insisted. She wants you to know that her daughter loved to sing. Will you call her Sur in your book?' I said of course I would, and Ravi went on recounting his sister's life.

After a year, the family started asking why there was no child. This was a common situation, one I'd heard again and again from various women in different countries. Sometimes the grace period was as long as two or three years, but the pattern seemed to be the same. If a couple had not made a baby, then either they weren't trying hard enough or there was something wrong with the wife. Lakshman's family reacted differently from many others, though. They organized a short break for the couple: four days in a region that was famed for its beauty, so they might have time to relax in each other's company. The intention was very clear: free from domestic and work responsibilities, they would have lots of sex and a child would be sure to appear.

Bhakti described these days as the last time that her daughter was truly happy. When she returned, she too seemed sure she was pregnant and when her usually regular period was late, she immediately shared the news with her family. But a week later she began to bleed and Lakshman, the gentle man whom she had loved since childhood, hit her for the first time. She didn't tell Bhakti, not then, but later, after there had been several more slaps and she had a cut on her arm from where one of his rings had broken her skin.

'My sister didn't blame Lakshman, you know. She just hated herself. She did grow to hate his parents, though, because they were always getting at her, mocking her, saying she was like a parched land. Sur was sure that Lakshman hit her because his parents expected him to do so. It was her punishment, something to make her try harder. My sister was ten years older than me. Now I'm the age she was then, but, unlike her, I've been to university. It's inconceivable to me that no one thought that perhaps there was a medical problem with Lakshman.'

Sur's in-laws sent her to doctors and clinics who said simply, give it time. To Bhakti's knowledge, no one suggested that Lakshman be tested. When three years had passed without change, his family took a different approach. Ravi told me how Sur's in-laws arranged for her and Lakshman to travel to the Gajapati district in the state of Odisha. 'In this place, there is a cannon. It's old, and many local Hindus believe it is a fertility shrine.'

The cannon was installed by the British Army in 1840 in the Rayagada Block of Gajapati and is half-buried on a hill, surrounded by thick forest, shaded by the fern-shaped leaves of neem trees. On a recent trip to India, I went to find it. There isn't a temple or even a shrine, but I watched dozens of locals follow the narrow, winding path that has been cleared through the trees, carrying coconuts, bananas and incense, to gather around the cannon and say prayers. Immersed in the heady scent of the burning sticks and the chattering cries and songs of the birds, I imagined Sur and Lakshman, who came during the Hindu month of Chaitra, when the cannon becomes a place of pilgrimage for the childless, rather than just an auspicious site. The hopeful believe that by pouring some milk into a small hole at the top of the cannon a child may be conceived.

Sur and Lakshman followed this path, through the dense, vibrant, living, cacophonous green, carrying some milk in a bottle or a jar. I assume it was Sur who poured the milk into the cannon; after all, they both believed it was she who was in some way cursed. I wonder how they felt when they left. Hopeful for a child, of course, but did Sur also think

longingly of the easiness and love of her relationship before
all the futility of their trying? Was her prayer, her puja, that
her husband would love her again, once a child was born?

Ravi told me that Sur returned, shining, from the shrine.
Bhakti nodded, as if she understood, and then spoke quickly
to her son, almost interrupting him. 'It didn't last, though,
not even a day and a night. Her period started the evening
after she arrived home.' Ravi was matter-of-fact, interpreting like a professional. He is a business man and probably
felt awkward discussing his sister's menstrual cycle, yet he
related each part of the story unflinchingly, even gracefully,
with careful, almost old-fashioned formality.

The narrative seemed to have a momentum of its own. I
knew the sad outcome, because the person who had put us
in touch had intimated it to me, but I had not discussed it
with Bhakti and Ravi. I didn't know if they knew that I was
aware of it. Instead they recounted events as they unfolded:
a tale of beatings and abuse, heard through neighbours and
relatives who lived in the same village as Sur and Lakshman,
because Sur no longer came to visit her own family and,
when they tried to see her, they were turned away, told she
was too busy for company. But there were rumours. Stories
of a bruised eye that took over a week to turn yellow, and
of shouting in the evening. No one did anything. She was
barren. It was awful for Lakshman's family. If there was
sympathy, it was mostly for them, not for the woman whose
failure to conceive had brought this upon herself.

Between the two villages, there is dense, tangled forest,
very similar to the area around the sacred cannon, and here
too there are neems, those hardiest of trees that need little
water to survive and only lose their leaves in the very worst

of droughts. Late one night, just over four months after they returned from offering milk to the cannon, after four cycles of disappointment, Sur climbed up a neem tree on the edge of the woods with a length of rope. In the morning, as the village came to life, they found her hanging there, dressed in a pale-blue sari, her bodily fluids already dried on the ground beneath her.

Bhakti lost her composure as she described that last fateful scene, weeping softly, but Ravi did not. He spoke almost in anger. I had been haunted by the women of the newspaper reports, had dreamt more than once of their falling and their burning. Now I felt in this sad, slow recounting over a broadband connection that I had known one of them: Sur, the girl who liked to sing, who loved and married her childhood sweetheart, and who took her life because she couldn't have a baby of her own.

But it wasn't the end of our conversation. From the folds of her sari, Bhakti produced a photograph and held it up. A girl in a red silk wedding sari smiled at me. Ravi said, 'My sister.' And then he added, 'For us, you know, suicide is not just despair; she will have hoped that in the next life she would be fertile, have many babies.'

Those Who Long:
Castigation and Stigmatization

Sur's story came to me unexpectedly, like a rumour or a whisper might, but meanwhile I had made contact with a charity called Reach India, which aims to bring 'training and other services to poor girls, women and the organizations that serve them, so they might empower girls and women to make positive changes in their lives, families and communities'[18] From its origins in 2007, it has supported communities with health advice, financial planning and educational programmes. One of the charity's great strengths is that it works closely with women and girls in regions its support workers know well and where they are trusted; they operate both in urban slums in Calcutta and in remote, rural areas. While the stigmatization and abuse of childless women is not Reach India's primary concern, its CEO, Partha Rudra, does see it as a key issue and one that is addressed very little at present.

The charity offered me unique access to women in rural and remote areas, who are the most likely to suffer from the stigma that childlessness can bring. I came to hear testament of the castigation and cruelty that is suffered so widely by infertile girls and women in India. While men may suffer psychologically as a result of not becoming fathers, in the patriarchal societies of India and south-east Asia, women are invariably blamed and often beaten for childlessness in a couple. Part of a vicious circle, this type of male violence may be seen as a way to perpetuate and re-establish men's hegemony: 'The inability to have a child makes a man emasculated; he reasserts his dominant position by subjugating his wife through physical pain.'[19]

The stories came to me piecemeal, in instalments. The field worker, Priyanka, travelled in remote regions and I had to wait until she encountered and re-encountered each of the subjects in the course of her duties. But short, heart-rending summaries, ending with tantalizing sentences, grew into vignettes. And although they were often translated into broken English, the grammar somehow represented the state of the speaker better than a more prescriptively correct syntax ever could.

There were interpreted stories where the meaning was unclear yet still imaginable in its awfulness. The sentence 'She attempted to conceive many times but the ovary got aborted' left me with illogical images of an empty ovary in a jar, like a Victorian relic. Not an embryo – a foetus in formaldehyde, which would itself somehow denote fertility rather than its opposite – but a sack without eggs, aborted because it had no function.

Through snippets of background information and Priyanka's careful transcriptions of her conversations, interspersed with local lore, the biographies of three women gradually emerged. One had a happy ending, but another told of a life that, in one of the brightest, most colourful countries on the planet, had had all the light taken out of it.

Saharbanu is forty-five and lives in the Murshidabad district in West Bengal. Married at twelve, by nineteen she longed to have a baby of her own. Like the other families in their village, she and her husband, Mr Robiulsk, lived in extreme poverty, but, despite that, Saharbanu recalls 'quality time' spent with her husband in those first years. He was a loving man, five years her senior, and she was happy to be with him. She lived with her in-laws and found them kind in those halcyon, early times. But as one, then two, then more years passed without a pregnancy, the relationship grew strained and the couple turned to a local travelling doctor, whom Saharbanu describes as a 'quack'. Financial constraints as well as a lack of awareness of what medical help might be available meant that they never approached a qualified medic or visited the district hospital, but instead relied on potions concocted by the itinerant medicine man, believing his pronouncement that if they did not work, it was because Saharbanu could never have a child.

Mr Robiulsk had always worked as a day labourer locally, but as the disdain of the village towards his wife grew, so it seemed did his, and he took work that was further and further away, so he saw Saharbanu only occasionally. Saharbanu, a Muslim, nevertheless took to visiting Hindu temples to pray that she might have a child. Manasa is a popular Hindu goddess in Bengal, often asked to bless a marriage or end childlessness. Usually pictured entwined with snakes, she is frequently unhappy and angry at being rejected by her husband and her father, Shiva, and hated by her stepmother, Chandra. It was not difficult to imagine a young woman in Saharbanu's position turning to a goddess whose own life was as troubled as her own, but who had the power to change things. Such visits were forbidden by Islamic law, seen as *haram*, but her husband, perhaps because they offered him hope, did not prevent them or even speak against them.

When Saharbanu's periods stopped with the advent of the menopause, she gave up even this last attempt at intervention. Now, she is abused by neighbours, family and former friends as *banja*, a woman who cannot conceive, and although her in-laws are still polite to her face, they abuse her to others when she is not there. Her husband no longer supports her financially and so she has turned to the bidi industry. Bidis are traditional cigarettes, handmade by rolling sun-dried tobacco into a tendu leaf. The work is highly skilled, with each worker rolling between 500 and 1,000 cigarettes a day, and popular among poor rural women and children who work from home. But it is also dangerous, with medical reports confirming the high carcinogenic risk as well as cases of tuberculosis and gynaecological and musculoskeletal conditions.[20]

Saharbanu's last words about her life now is that she is 'spending her life in darkness and never participates in any occasions'.

Bharti Devi was wed to Dihendra when she was seventeen and lived in a house that was half-mud, half-cement with her in-laws, who also, at first, treated her kindly. But while Bharti did conceive, again and again, the children did not stay in her womb, and with each miscarriage the kindness and support of her husband's family diminished. Turning to their son, they urged him to take a second wife, but Dihendra refused, defying them. With the help of a local group, the couple learned about adoption and were successful in legally adopting a one-day-old boy. With the advent of her son, Bharti's life once again changed. Welcomed anew by her in-laws, reassured by her husband, she rejoices that 'she again starts to live her life fully'.

Of all the narratives I heard, Bharti's story was the only one that ended well. There were small but important differences. She had actually conceived. Her husband loved his wife enough to defy his parents in the face of convention. There was a local self-help group with the knowledge and financial resources to show them how to legally adopt a child. And there was a final thing, less obvious perhaps: Bharti was pleased that she was again welcomed by her husband's family. Her capacity to forgive their eagerness to push her aside, their treatment of her during her childlessness, was warm and magnanimous, illuminating the life she had yet to live with her reconciled husband and her son.

The final story was that of Ratho, who is twenty-eight. What was unusual about her story was not her childlessness but her husband's alcoholism; he beat her frequently and there was not enough money for necessities because he spent it on his addiction. Ratho sees her own childlessness as worsening the addiction somehow, literally driving her husband to drink more and more. Her husband's brother was also violent. It was not until Ratho's mother-in-law was moved by the plight of her other daughter-in-law, the one who was not childless, that she acknowledged the pain of the young women who lived with her. Ratho joined a self-health group run by a local charity, but when members spoke to her husband about his increasing violence, she asked them to stop lest it make the situation worse. However, the group has given her some independence; she makes jelly and jam and saves in the hope of finding treatment for her infertility.

This sketch of her life was marked by Ratho's determination to take on blame. My husband is an alcoholic *because I am childless*; my husband hits me *because I am childless*; she believes that, through working, the treasure she will gain is not more independence or freedom from her husband, but treatment for the problem that she perceives as *her fault*. Her utter faith that the solution lies within her reach, that she alone can make her world right again, by giving birth to a baby that will restore her standing and redeem her husband, can be seen as empowering. Or it may be that the alternatives – leaving him or being abandoned, cast out from her family, without even the possibility of a baby – were too bleak to contemplate.

Those Who Long: Afterwards

In some cultures the repercussions of childlessness and infertility are so great that only denying their actuality can make your prospects imaginable, but in others a diagnosis is the beginning of a difficult journey towards an unplanned future. The realization that current scientific advances cannot help you does not bring an end to longing. Instead your yearning becomes a persistent, discomfiting thing, very occasionally forgotten, but made more painful on its return by the brief respite.

Kate, a thirty-five-year-old driving instructor from Wales, spoke to me of how acceptance of her inability to have a child eluded her for years. 'After the full hysterectomy, Eric and I knew logically we wouldn't have birth children of our own, but it was three, maybe four, years before I stopped having those thoughts – you know, when you pass children's clothing and see a cute dress, and think, I'll get that for my daughter when I have one, or you see an ad for a new kid's film and think about taking your yet-to-be-born children to the pictures. No sooner did I think those things than a horrible voice in my head would say, Stop this, it's not going to happen, don't be ridiculous. I even cried in the middle of Monsoon once, looking at the children's clothing section.'

Mardy Ireland's book *Reconceiving Women: Separating Motherhood from Female Identity* discusses women who strongly identify with a stereotypical female gender role identity. Women, who, like Kate, have said yes to a child but have been let down by their bodies can be the most vulnerable to any negative comments about their lack of children. In Ireland's view, 'The central issue among these women is one of mourning. They must grieve the real loss of their physical integrity, the loss of their anticipated child, and the loss of their imagined identities as mothers.'[21] Missing something that has never happened, but has always seemed inevitable, that is inextricably tied to your sense of self, must be mourned and grieved for. Ireland goes on to suggest that the longer you have tried to get pregnant unsuccessfully, the longer the mourning period you may need. It is as if each disappointment, each failure – because we all too often see it as a lack in ourselves – begins a period of renewed mourning. Only when the treatment is over, and the diagnosis accepted, can true mourning begin, and with it the hope of acceptance.

Charisse, who comes from south-west Nigeria, emailed me about her personal experience of unsuccessful IVF. Charisse is Yoruba and among this large ethnic group childlessness has its own social meaning. Upon marriage, a wife becomes a 'visitor' rather than a full member of her husband's patrilineage. Children born into the family consolidate its status and perpetuity, so a childless woman has no value to the family she has married into. Historically, a childless Yoruba woman would not be buried but instead her body left in the open for wild animals to devour. The stigma remains in the culture and because childbearing, as in so many other cultures, is regarded an essential step to adulthood, an infertile woman can never be respected as a peer by other adults and is denied a voice.[22] In her article on the stigma of childlessness among the Yoruba, Tola Pearce cites a forty-year-old woman who 'won't have the privilege of voicing her opinion in public, as she might wish'.[23]

Charisse described her in-laws as 'very progressive' and said she had been 'very lucky in many respects', so she had never felt the shame and ostracism that she had seen other women experience. However, she did feel that there was a strong cultural bias towards childbearing and childrearing and that to choose not to have children was not even a possibility. Her biggest worry was that her doctors were unable to find any medical reason why she and her husband should not conceive. After five rounds of gruelling IVF, they gave up. But Charisse's email was a positive one. She was keen to share her story, because, despite what she described as a 'period of black', she went on to find happiness and fulfilment in a new career as a journalist. She still wished that she had been a mother, but now she also questioned whether she had been conditioned to want that: 'It's not that I stopped wishing I could have been a mom, but that I wonder why I had always assumed that was the only thing I could be. I'm happy in my life now, I love my husband and my work, and I'm a little sorry for all those years we spent chasing something that really wasn't meant to be for me. I'm a very different person now.'

For Charisse, her failure to conceive opened up an opportunity that she hadn't even considered could be part of her future: that of a successful woman in a professional field. For one of Ireland's subjects, the realization that she could separate her identity as a woman from her child-lessness came from gaining a feminist perspective rather than finding a fulfilling career. Feminism enabled her to see her life as a different thing, defined more by who she was than by a role that was expected of her but which she could never assume.

Jo, from Australia, found a different way of dealing with her childlessness, which is in marked contrast to those men and women who surround themselves with the children of friends and family to lessen their pain. She and her husband had resorted to IVF without success, taking the decision to give up on it only when they felt they were both too old responsibly to be parents any more. Jo's work as a teacher means she is surrounded by children every day, while her husband, the son of a midwife, runs the local shop in their very small Australian town, and deals constantly with mums and their children doing the family shop. Jo's town has seen a recent baby boom, with four or five children per family as the norm, but for both Jo and her husband being around children is a painful experience that serves only to highlight their own loss. 'People's attitudes have been surprising. We decided early on to have a line. If asked if we had children . . . we decided to say that we couldn't, "which was very upsetting" and that "we'd leave it there" – effectively cutting off the conversation. We also don't allow babies in our home, because it's our refuge, but we are softening up to having the child of close friends. Everyone responded to this. Word got around. Unless someone is new to town, people don't talk about babies or kids around us.'

One of the hardest things for Jo is seeing children whose parents do not look after them well, or at all: 'I find parent–teacher interviews excruciating, because so many parents do a lacklustre job of raising their children. We both struggle with parents of unwanted children of any form – we're incredibly judgemental, and it helps to be unapologetic about this between ourselves.'

Despite her forthrightness, as a teacher Jo is still subject to comments about how a childless person doesn't understand children: 'I used to (and sometimes still do) regularly get stick from parents of students when I had to ring them about some kind of misdemeanour or issue at school. They would often throw out the comment that 'You wouldn't understand this because you don't have children . . .' until I learnt to approach all such conversations with a quick affirmation that parenting is hard and say something that made them feel as though I didn't think they were bad parents. Now that I am approaching fifty, I don't get it as much, but young teachers experience this kind of comment a lot and it magically disappears when they have their own children. It's like they have been accepted into the club.'

Jo's upbringing in Adelaide seemed more anonymous than her current lifestyle. She notes that newly married women once again tend to take their husband's name, something that was less common when she was young, and observes that two young women she works with feel alienated from their peer group because they have not yet fallen pregnant. Jo felt the city was safer somehow, and keeping her maiden name made her feel that she had 'privacy, a nomenclature buffer, a critical distance of surname'.[24] The friendliness of the small town where she now lives is as much a drawback as an advantage, because it so often seems 'there is nowhere to hide'.

Those Who Long: Childless by Circumstance

These are the women and men who end up being childless simply because it is how their life has turned out. Perhaps they found a partner too late for it to be physically possible for them to have a baby, or maybe they never found someone at all; their period of longing for a child is just beginning as other people are learning to adjust.

The writer Melanie Notkin suggests that rather than the career-focussed women portrayed in the media as 'too self-centered and too selfish for motherhood', many childless women just want to be in a committed relationship before having children and never meet the right partner for this to be possible. Or if they do find a life partner, they do so when it is too late for them to have biological children. In 2012 a *Time Magazine* cover story, 'The Childfree Life: When Having It All Means Not Having Children', correlated the decreasing American birth rate with more people choosing to be childless, yet Notkin notes that, according to the author of a National Health Statistics report into fertility in the United States, only 14 per cent of all childless women are voluntarily so. For the others, their lack of offspring is often 'exacerbated by the inexhaustible myth' that they have chosen not to be mothers.[25]

The problems of forming a lasting relationship and of having a successful career can seem inextricably linked. Notkin cites the case of Joanna, a thirty-eight-year-old attorney, who left the partner track to move to a less demanding role 'in order to attract men who did not find her profession competitive with theirs'. Joanna regrets her choice, feeling 'heartbroken that I'm still single and not a mom. I regret taking a major step down in my career.'

Valerie is a forty-five-year-old architect from New York state. When she contacted me via social media, she immediately volunteered that she had always wanted children, and her life plan had been that by thirty or so she would be in a settled relationship or married and then a family would follow. 'But it just didn't happen. I went through a period of ill-advised sexual encounters, and each time I hoped it was going to lead to something more. It wasn't the men, it was me. I was trying too hard.'

By her mid-thirties, Valerie, still single, toyed with the idea of having a child with a donor. A friend, Jas, had offered to donate his sperm and she seriously considered single motherhood. 'But it wasn't for me. I just couldn't see how I could do it all – my work, the nappies, the child care – without someone to support me. And then I worried about Jas's role. Would he be a father? Or just a donor? He said he was open to parenting, but it seemed odd and untraditional somehow. I really wanted a wedding and picket fence and turn-taking for night feeds. I didn't want to be a single mom. God knows, I'd been careful enough with contraception over the years to prevent it.'

Then last year, at her forty-fourth birthday party, Valerie met someone. Dave moved in with her six months later and she spoke about her certainty that he was the one. But Dave is sixty and feels too old to start a family. 'I accept it, of course I do,' Valerie said. 'I even think he's right, and maybe I'm too old now too, but, of course, I'm sorry for how it is, and sad.'

Writing in the *Guardian*, Bibi Lynch railed against the way mothers so often do not seem to appreciate having the thing that she most wished for.[26] She explains that she 'simply never met the right man' and speaks of her regret at not knowing the love between mother and child, the one 'that finally makes sense of our existence'. The agony of knowing she won't experience motherhood is such that she realizes she would 'change every decision I ever made that led me to this place'. In a follow-up article, written over four years later, Lynch, still grieving, has found that the pain of being childless is not the worst she has to deal with. Rather, 'not having kids means I mean nothing in our society. And I never really saw that devastating PS coming.'[27]

Lynch describes how on the *Victoria Derbyshire* show on BBC Two, the television presenter introduced the aunt of Aylan Kurdi, the Syrian refugee child who drowned in the Mediterranean while trying to reach a new life with his father, by saying, 'If you're a parent, you might find this upsetting.' I saw that broadcast too and, like Lynch, I was incensed that anyone could be so narrow-minded, so utterly lacking in empathy, as to suppose that a necessary condition of being moved by a dead child was to have borne one yourself.

It was as if, for all of us – the involuntarily childless – the sadness of our state, the missing out on something longed for, marked us as deficient, not just in our biology, in our ability to make good choices or to find the right partner, but in our very being. Because we do not, or cannot, have children, we are branded as less caring, less kind, and consequently of less value.

Derbyshire's thoughtless delimiting wasn't the far more heinous societal exclusion of the Indian women, the expected physical violence of a disappointed husband, or the *huis clos* of Noor living with her husband and his second wife. But in a twenty-first-century society that is supposedly gender equal and believes itself to be inherently just, the casual nature of the remark was a potent reminder of how unsympathetic, how callous, how different, other people still sometimes perceive us to be.

A Short Note about Love

My husband is childless because I am. Yet when we met, the intention to have children was something we agreed on from the very beginning. It's a difficult thing, that navigation in the early days of a relationship. Mentioning children hints at a commitment that one or both of you may not feel ready for. Avoiding it until your future together seems irrevocable can lead to a lifetime of regret, of unspoken blame, of disappointment, even resentment.

We were lucky – if, in retrospect, you can call it that. The subject of children came up a few months after we had started seeing each other, in the guarded way that must be typical among many couples – if you settle down one day, will you have children? It was an easy question for both of us; we both said yes, and that was that. Or not. I wasn't a good bet – I even said something like that to Alan in those early days, when my endometriosis had not been diagnosed but I suffered excruciating period pain. On our second date, I passed out after a pub lunch only to come round to see him beside me, looking worried, but embroiled in an argument with someone who had sneered that it was disgusting to see someone so drunk this early in the day. I hadn't drunk any alcohol at all; I was taking strong painkillers, which precluded it. In the battle between my oozing, battered body and the medication, the former had had a brief victory and the shock of the pain – something even now, so

many, many years later – I cringe to recall, had sent me into
unconsciousness.

At the time my GP's explanation was that some women
have painful periods; take some pills. It was only when we
started to try to have a child that a battery of tests showed
that I had endometriosis, which causes inner bleeding.
Every month, for years, my body had had its own internal
menstruation of a kind, in various anatomical places, with
differing degrees of damage. Endometriosis is common
enough, you learn, once you know what it is, but occurs
with widely varying degrees of severity. Mine was severe
but, in my stubbornness, I adamantly refused to have a
hysterectomy. That, it seemed to me, would end even the
possibility of hope, even if it did bring respite from the pain.

Instead there were surgeries to tidy up, make a little more
space, a little less mess. And through them all, Alan, cleaning
my post-surgical wounds, calling from work every other hour
to see how I was. Once, when we'd taken a weekend break
away from it all, he had to run around Budapest trying to
find me sanitary towels late in the evening while I lay in
bed with bundles of toilet paper stuffed between my legs,
wondering if the internal bleeding had also decided to come
after ten days instead of twenty-eight this month.

Amidst it all, we found a camaraderie – it was us against
it, whatever the outcome. And when early menopause
brought an end to all that bleeding, we agreed that we were
indeed fortunate, because for a few women even that does
not bring a cessation of the internal cycle. Occasionally we
would share our sadness that we didn't have children, but
much less so than we had done when we had waged our war
against my body. Mostly we had a quiet rejoicing. We could

go on holiday together without having to take into account my unpredictable cycle, knowing that a much needed one-week summer break would no longer turn into a week of me crying in bed, or passing out in unexpected places when I did venture to leave the hotel room. We travelled because we could. I had taken to doing contract work during the worst years of my illness, because it was easier to manage a few hours a day, no matter what my body was doing, and I hated to let anyone down. But now, post-menopause, post-pain, I took on more and more work and eventually got a permanent job teaching at a university again. I had missed the fellowship of a department, the witnessing of young lives unfolding over three years of study, the challenge of work-ing with brilliant, demanding postgraduates. The university work, coupled with my publishing contracts, was unfettered by regular days of immobility and sickness. We moved around a lot – in one five-year period we lived in three countries and worked in four – and by the time we returned home to London, it was as if we were taking up a different life. Yes, it was one without children, and we had taken time to adjust to that, but it was also a freer one than I had known for years.

But pain has memories. I can't walk around Islington in north London without thinking of the cab that brought us home after one of my operations. How the speed bumps, each and every one of them, made me cry out, and how my husband held me, asking the driver again and again to try and be as gentle as he could.

We lived in Liguria, in Italy, for three years, and one of my most powerful recollections is of the doctor and two nurses, all women, who kindly, spontaneously, gathered round me in an awkward group hug after looking at a particularly gruesome scan of my damaged insides, because they thought it must be awful to know that I would never have a child. Their empathy was moving but also strengthening, because I was being embraced, not rejected. That's how it was for me with Alan too. Our solidarity in the face of shared adversity gave me potency because there was always somewhere I belonged, and that place was our relationship.

Robert Frost ends his poem *Hyla Brook* with the line: 'We love the things we love for what they are.'[1]

I believe that even my brokenness was loved because it was part of me. When I look at my husband, every day, even after the occasional fierce argument, I can never forget the steadfast kindness, the loyalty, the love, that brought us both through all of this.

A Short Note on Bleeding

I have not had endometriosis for almost ten years now. Yet still the viscosity and colour of accidental blood affects me.

I wait in a queue for a public toilet and when I enter the cubicle I find the woman before me has left a thin trail of blood down the side of the pan. It is bright red, running and I try to remember the woman who came out. Did she seem to be in pain?

This is how the memory of the constant irregularity of pain remains – irregularity because the twenty-eight-day cycle that should have made the debilitating days predictable could be anything from ten to thirty-two; constant because, between the acute pain of menstruation, there was an interminable dull throb, a physical memory of what had gone before, and a reminder of what awaited me.

'Debilitating days' isn't quite the right phrase. It's not that there were days when I felt 'weak and infirm'. That sounds too passive somehow. They were howling, screaming days; the only quiet times were when I passed out – in the middle of a supermarket, after Sunday lunch, once while giving a lecture. If my period was early and completely unexpected, the pain could come on suddenly. And I would find myself on the floor crying, rolled in a ball, perhaps howling for it to stop, or retching on my knees.

Ten per cent of women worldwide have endometriosis

and within that group as many as 30 to 50 per cent will be infertile. It is the second most common gynaecological condition, but it took my GP no less than seven crucial, fertility-changing years to refer me for the tests needed to diagnose it.

There were drugs for the pain of course, which only took an hour or so to work – pills that left me feeling muffled, as if my head was filled with something that deadened not just the pain receptors but my brain too. They made me queasy, gave me chronic diarrhoea, and therefore defeated the other reason for taking them, apart from pain relief: to allow me to work, to go out, to do something, to keep busy, to stop all my thoughts being focussed on how many days this time; how long will my period last?

Thick clots of blood laced with black that defeated every kind of sanitary towel. A lumpy mess, glutinous as a miscarriage, as an almost-conceived thing. Eventually, after diagnosis, I understood, finally, that the pain was because it was not just my uterus that was bleeding. Layers of congealed stickiness joining my organs together, pulling on them whenever I moved, or even if I didn't. I was disgusted by my own bodily function

And oh, what that bleeding paid for.

It was the price of my thick, shining hair and unlined skin, of youthfulness. It might have been the price of a child, had it not made me infertile. In my early forties, my periods stopped. A sympathetic doctor in Doha spoke to me about the menopause, gently, I think, expecting tears. I already knew I couldn't have children; all I felt at this new revelation was relief. Suddenly the years stretched out before me. I had not had a hysterectomy even after I knew pregnancy was an impossibility, because I was counting on an early menopause just like my mother, and here it was. There was occasional bleeding, twice in that last year, but much less disruptive, and brief – just four days instead of my usual eight to ten. I thought then, in saying goodbye to this thing – this malevolent, messy recalcitrance that I had carried round inside me for more than two decades – that perhaps this was what it would have been like to be a healthy young woman.

And yes, of course, that would have been a good thing to be. But relief outweighs regret. I have not had endometriosis for almost ten years now, and I know how fortunate that makes me.

2

Those Who Believe

I am from a casually superstitious family. We throw salt over our shoulder, never leave a hat on a bed or shoes on a table. When my husband first met me, it amused him, but now he observes my superstitions too – touches wood, doesn't look at a full moon through glass but opens the window or the door. I don't really in my heart of hearts believe that these acts will somehow protect me, although I do think, oddly, that they can't do any harm. Was I somehow not fated to have children? Was there something that could have been done, some as-yet unknown act of atonement that might have reversed the limited possibilities of my body? Should I have left under my bed unswept and untidied, danced in the moon, never sat on that stone wall?[1] If it was not meant to be, then 'meant' by whom or what?

Superstitious belief is a Janus: it may offer hope when all else fails or is out of reach, but it can also lead to condemnation and revilement.

In the first year following the news of my infertility, I developed a tendency that flew in the face of my usual scholarly rigour: I searched myriad sources, many with very little exactitude to commend them, for information about my condition. I have long red hair. Three medical 'cross-sectional' studies suggested a correlation between endometriosis and red hair. Other papers dismissed these finds as rubbish.

For me, it was a temporary fascination, which settled into a practical evaluation of my position. We could adopt, but did we want to? Or we could live a life without children and instead find pleasure in the children of our friends. For many others, in part because of culture or predisposition, this shift would never occur. In Qatar, Noor continued to hope for a miracle from Allah; other women and some men in different countries looked for it in strange places, in quiet prayers and blessings, or penitential actions whose rituals seemed eternally caught between the suffering of punishment and the hope of reward.

Those Who Believe: Prayers

One February, long after we had acknowledged that we would never have a child, my husband and I travelled to Naples. I was researching a novel there and in the chaotic decaying splendour of the old Spanish Quarter we noticed a queue of people standing outside a small chapel. We hesitated and looked. An unobtrusive sign said that it was the Church of Saint Mary Frances of the Five Wounds of Christ. Above the church was her eighteenth-century home.

At the age of sixteen, Mary Frances joined the Third Order of St Francis and spent half of her life in that house, sleeping on the first floor with another nun, while the priest who owned the building slept in a room above them. She was born in Naples and became a nun to avoid being forced into marriage by her abusive father. Her years, so the story went, had been spent in physical and mental trials, with visitations from the Angel Raphael and stigmata on her hands, which she wore gloves to conceal.[2] The first saint to be canonized in Naples, Mary Frances was well loved throughout the city, but especially in the Spanish Quarter, which named her their patron saint and celebrates her feast day on 6 October every year. Strangely, the shrine of this saint, whose life was known for its hardship and chastity was now achieving fame throughout Italy as a place where the childless may be blessed with a baby.

We joined the queue, a long snaking line of heterosexual couples that wound through the narrow doorway and along the street past two other doors. It was a restless line. Many people left for a few minutes, to squeeze past those waiting at the door, to say a prayer in the chapel to the side or to light a candle there. The atmosphere was incongruous for a church; there was the kind of expectancy you find before a concert or a show starring a celebrity you admire. People murmured attestations to each other. Sometimes I struggled to understand anything at all, but some of the visitors were clearly from northern Italy, where we had lived for some years, and I eavesdropped on their stories, hastily whispering translations to my husband. A cousin had fallen pregnant only one month after sitting in the chair, after four years of fertility treatment; another woman had borne a child even though her periods had stopped almost two years before. This was a queue of hope. We were not there because we believed that Saint Mary Frances would intervene for us. I was there out of curiosity. The queue continued up a long staircase. In the upstairs room were relics and historical artefacts of the saint, amongst them a chair – an old wooden armchair, covered in a woollen blanket: the miracle chair. Men and women would sit on it to be blessed by the attendant nuns. The walls of the first room were covered in cards of thanks and baby cards, but there was also one of Saint Mary Frances's hair shirts and the whip she would beat herself with in penance. At first we were unsure whether to leave the queue, since we had reached the rooms themselves. I vacillated, feeling somehow fraudulent because I'm not a Catholic, yet longing to have the experience. We now thought ourselves too set in the life that we had made – too old, in truth – to start having children of our own, even if some miracle were possible, but that did not mean we had forgotten how it felt to long. And there was something in that small space, those hopeful crowds, that touched me, although, unusually for me, I could not find the words to explain to my husband why it was so.

A dear friend of mine, an Italian and a devout Catholic, had been struggling to have a baby for some time, so I resolved to take the blessing for her sake. I reasoned with my husband, whispering, that if I told her I had done so, and sent a prayer card from the shrine to Japan, where she now lived, it might give her some comfort, some more hope. It certainly could do no harm. My husband, an inveterate non-believer, surprised me, because when our turn came, he too sat on the chair and consented to the blessing, I think out of fondness for our friend, but also a kind of solidarity. An elderly nun touched each of us with a wooden cross as we sat on the chair. Following the example of those before us, we whispered Amen, and, for some reason I can't quite understand, I also said, '*Grazie*,' which made my husband smile a little.

I waited at the sales counter, feeling somewhat cynical

about the sale of religious items. But it was quickly dispelled by the nun's kindness when I explained I wanted something to send to a friend who hoped for a child; she gave me two little prayer cards for free in addition to the lace one that I paid a tiny, insignificant sum for. We left, went out into the narrow Neapolitan street, where the sky was just a thin ribbon of blue and the air was filled with the smell of garlic, tomatoes and olive oil, and walked hand in hand to a nearby trattoria without saying anything at all. Had I been of an age to hope, I know that I would for a time have felt changed by it somehow, as if, mysteriously, something might be possible again, but now I thought only of my friend. She received the prayer delightedly. Almost a year later she gave birth to a daughter.

Christian hagiography is replete with stories involving conception and birth. There is Saint Anne, mother of the Virgin Mary, who after almost five decades of infertility was miraculously blessed with a baby much later in life than would be possible without modern scientific intervention. There is Saint Gianna Beretta Molla, who sacrificed her own life for the child she gave birth to, and there are other saints, like Saint Mary Frances, whose relics and shrines are believed to make the childless conceive. One of the most famous is an icon in the Church of Panagia on the island of Tinos in Greece.[3]

In the sweltering heat of summer, on the day of the Assumption of the Virgin, 15 August, every year women can be seen crawling on their hands and knees from the port, where the tourists and traders arrive on ferries and boats, over a kilometre uphill, to the white grandiosity of the church. Pelagia, an octogenarian nun, found an icon of the virgin there in 1823 and the church was built to honour the site. Within the church the shrine awaits, its miracles related and attested to by the faithful; for them it is a bringer of birth to those who believe themselves to be infertile. When we arrived, the day before the pilgrimage, the heat was intense and reminded me of Qatar. The church's whiteness shimmered in the light as people went about their day-to-day business, but early the following morning it was already possible to see the expectant, hopeful pilgrims. They were mostly women. In the course of the day I saw only one man, young and dark-skinned, crawling towards the church. One middle-aged woman wore traditional Indian dress and while the steps leading up to the church were covered in worn carpet, the pavement leading from the port to the stairs had torn her fine silk sari. Other women wore jeans and T-shirts, which seemed anachronistic somehow, given the ritual they performed. And of course there were local women, or at least from elsewhere in Greece, clad in modest black dresses with headscarves tied under their chin. I assumed they were older, perhaps nearing menopause, but then a headscarf slipped and the woman halted, kneeling back to refasten it, and I saw that she was no more than twenty-five or so.

I had no wish to disturb women enacting a ritual that they believed could change their life, but in the evening I spoke to the woman who owned the taverna where I was staying and she promised to introduce me to her cousin, who could speak English and had made the pilgrimage five years ago and now had a daughter, named Pelagia, for the saint who had granted her heart's wish.

Evi was tiny and looked very young. I imagined her on her knees crawling towards the icon and thought that five years ago she must have been little older than a child. 'I was twenty,' she said, 'and we had been trying for a baby for two years since we were married. Doctors told me I had polycystic ovaries, but the drugs they gave me didn't seem to help.'

I asked if she knew anyone else who had made the pilgrimage and she said yes, but that not everyone was blessed. 'I think when I made the journey to ask for a child, it was just me showing that I believed God could grant me one if he so wished. Sometimes he doesn't choose to do so, because perhaps he sees a different path for that couple. We can't understand God, only try to have faith.'

We did not speak long; her sister was looking after Pelagia and Evi was on her way to collect her. But her quiet conviction, her faith that this was something that had been granted, rather than an act of biology, summed up the beliefs of those crawling, begging women I had watched the day before. I wondered if those who, unlike Evi, were not chosen felt as certain of the will of God as she did, or if their childlessness caused them to lose their faith.

Many people are resolute in their belief that observing their faith in a particular way has brought them a child. Churches and religious organizations offer a plethora of prayers and interventions for those who believe God might help them. I was, and am, wary of many such claims. While the generous kindness of the nuns had disarmed me in Naples, I remain sceptical and condemnatory of the exploitation that too often accompanies the demands of those who peddle fertility to desperate men and women as if they alone are privy to God's grace to give it.

'We will be having deliverance, which is the casting out
of unclean spirits, for those who believe that it may be
a demonic spirit hindering them from conceiving. Are
you troubled with nightmares, wet dreams, tormenting
thoughts, spirit-husband, spirit-wife, recurrent
miscarriages and/or barrenness? You may be the perfect
candidate for deliverance.'

Pregnancy by Faith[4]

Below the message was a picture, not a photograph, of a
small curly-haired boy wearing a golden crown. I was in-
trigued. This faith was about losing some evil within you
rather than about receiving a blessing that could change
your biological fortune.

It was in complete opposition to the Greek Orthodox
church, which explicitly reassures couples: 'A couple that is
infertile through no fault of their own is as loved by God,
His Church, and His people as anyone else. Involuntary
childlessness should never be equated with a curse, sin,
shame, or faithlessness.'[5]

Nevertheless, I could understand why someone might
believe in the concept of 'deliverance'; I empathized with
it. Before my early menopause, I had thought of my endo-
metrial lesions as malign inhabitants growing within me,
had imagined their sticky excretions as those of a parasitic
organism. It wasn't such a big step to visualize them as
wicked spirits that could be cast out. But still, it seemed to
place yet another burden on the infertile; here was something else that was wrong with them, something else that
needed to be healed. I wondered what the price might be,
in both monetary and emotional terms. Fertility and the

faithful is a lucrative business and a perpetual one. It ranges from the sale of relics in the medieval period to present-day advertisements for fertility bracelets, whose stones claim to help 'to stabilize hormonal changes such as PMS, PCOS and menopause'.

The website of Pregnancy by Faith displayed testimonies to the success of their ministry, with links to an online shop selling everything from books to anointing oil, fertility tea and T-shirts. The testimonials were joyful, expressing gratitude to the church; some included dismissive references to the failure of modern medical methods the writer had also tried, some with quite detailed accounts of their menstrual blood or the lack of it. Many mentioned the efficaciousness of a 'video prayer for supernatural conception'. This was free to listen to, on YouTube, preceded, bizarrely, by an advertisement for electricity. The opening picture was of an improbably muscular, bare-chested, winged man wearing a low-slung white girdle – a fantasy comic-strip angel. The prayer wasn't what I expected either. The promise of casting out demons that featured in the initial message had made me wary, but it was a succession of images: a rainbow, a picture of a compass that entreated you to 'Walk with Jesus', and again the super-hero angel. The words 'Supernatural Conception' would appear occasionally across the pictures, while the soundtrack was a woman speaking in a gentle voice, occasionally breaking into awkward song, and interspersing her prayer with halleluiahs and even laughter. It seemed like a gentle thing initially, a way to relax a believer, to stop them worrying about their inability to conceive, possibly medically beneficial in its ability to soothe.

But as the image changed to a baby's hand and the slogan

'Everything is Possible', so too did the tenet of the prayer: 'I command the devil to take his hands off of you.' Then a series of banishings: 'Depression', 'Confusion', 'Deep in Sorrow', all personified as evil spirits, and all cast away in Jesus's name. The demons were not sticky adhesions and damaged organs, but the sadness and despair such conditions could bring. Operations had tried to remove as much of mine as they could, but this was a cheap internet surgery of the soul.

I did not know I would be childless when I visited the Milk Grotto in Israel. It was the late 1990s and a temporary ceasefire in the hostilities meant that I could at last go. I travelled with a good friend, a childless man, who had no wish to become a father and who had in fact ended relationships with women over the very issue of parenthood. We planned to stay in kibbutzim for the most part and to travel to various religious sites as well as see the desert. The grotto was an accidental find. We saw it on a list of sites local to Bethlehem and found ourselves with time to spare. It's a cave hollowed out of soft white stone. The story is that Mary and Joseph, fleeing from Herod's murderous soldiers after an angel appeared to warn them of the slaughter which would cause the blood of children to fall about them like rain, stopped to feed their infant. A drop of Mary's breast milk fell, rendering the stone white and the place sacred. It was as if, I thought, the death of all those ancient children, their lost lives and grieving mothers, the wailing and loud lamentation, had somehow to be ameliorated in history by a story of hope, of life given where it might never have existed.

Since at least the fourth century people have been

worshipping here and they too, more than a thousand years ago, had come in hope. It is believed that by consuming a little of the powdered stone with food or drink, you may be blessed with a child. It's easy to mock, so we didn't, and even my smart-mouthed, cynical friend fell quiet in the softly pale glow of the vaulted walls. Was it the atmosphere, or perhaps the evidence of the grotto's successes – the plethora of letters in myriad tongues, the silent eloquence of photographs of newborns with their smiling parents? Women from as far afield as India, Argentina, the US, the Middle East and Europe had come to take a little of the soft white dust, to pray to Our Lady of Milk that they might be given a child. In this place the need to believe, the urgency of hope that something apart from biological childlessness might be in the years to come, acted as a broker of peace, as well as a survival mechanism. The Bethlehem cave, in all its simplicity, continues to be a destination for Muslims and Christians alike, a place of respite from the hostilities that surround it, a miracle as much in this coming together of ideologies as it is in the letters of gratitude for miraculous conceptions in Sri Lanka, in Spain, in Washington, in Dublin.

Those Who Believe and Suffer for It

Dehri is a small agricultural village in Uttar Pradesh, about 100 miles to the north of Delhi. Childless couples are regarded with suspicion, marked as cursed in a state known for its high birth rates, often forbidden from attending social and community events. Poverty is rife and the literacy rate below 60 per cent; most people lack much in the way of formal schooling and work in the fields to contribute to their family income as soon as they are able. Uttar Pradesh, the most populous state in India, is home to more than 8 per cent of the world's poor yet is only slightly larger than the United Kingdom. There, in the smallest of villages, and most destitute of towns, one group makes a good living: tantrics. They are regarded as holy men. In the West tantrism is best known and usually practised as a form of yoga originating from ancient mystical Hindu rituals, but the tantric wise men of India can belong to one of three religions: Buddhism, Islam or Hinduism. They are seen as spiritual interventionists, capable of communicating with supernatural powers and using them to improve earthly life. Some tantric rituals to bring about a change of fortune are benign and supportive of the adherent's need or wish, but there are also darker, terrifying practices.

Madan and Murti Simaru were desperate for a child.[6] Three years after their marriage, they turned to a local tantric with a reputation for helping with fertility problems. The first attempt, a talisman that Madan had to bury in the fields, did not lead to any change in their circumstances; on the second approach they were advised that a much greater ritual would be required. Monu Kumar was six, the child of a neighbour, not well known to them except as one of the many boys who played in the yards and alleyways. With the help of Murti's brother, the couple kidnapped the child one evening and took him to a mango grove just a few hundred metres from the village, on the banks of an irrigation canal.

It must have been a macabre night. The three villagers, the terrified six-year-old, the presiding tantric with his incantations and mantras. To the sound of his spells, Madan and Murti slowly killed the child while their relative watched. The police report does not give the details of the atrocity but it does state that by the end of the ceremony there was so much blood that Murti completed the ritual by bathing herself in it.

The perpetrators were caught and arrested. Madan and Murti's home, as well as that of Murti's brother, was torched to the ground by incensed neighbours. Yet Monu's father, Narendra Kumar, just twenty-two himself, spoke to the press, sitting in the small dried-clay courtyard outside his home of mud bricks. 'It is due to illiteracy and poverty that people get influenced by these tantrics,' he said, and appealed to the police to do more to eradicate the practices of the men who prey on such circumstances.

Local police spoke about their renewed attempts to end tantric human sacrifices following the murder in 2003. My informant said that tantrics were no longer welcome locally, whatever they promised or offered. Yet violent tantric practices continue, perhaps not in Dehri, but elsewhere in Uttar Pradesh, in Gujarat, in Andhra Pradesh, in Assam, in most of India. Tantrics promise wealth, fertility of a human being or fertility of the land, a charm against ill luck, power against the starvation and poverty that a bad harvest might bring. Most frequently reported is the selling of birds, rare owls and neelkanths, both protected by law, and peacocks, all with their wings fastened down, in some cases glued, their feet chopped off. They are sold to villagers who scrimp and save to sacrifice the helpless birds so they may be granted a wish. Uttar Pradesh is the hub of this trade in the flightless. For me these creatures are the antithesis of winged hope, but for others, for those who have no other means to escape the difficulties of their lives, they are a last remaining source of it.

As the economic gap widens between the agrarian poor, driven to despair and suicide by the growing costs of seed and rising debts, and much of urban India, tantrics offer a solution embedded in ancient superstition, the chimera of hope and a chance to gain control over a world that at times, for some, seems impossible to survive in.

'When a woman cannot have children, she is either a witch or a victim of witchcraft.'

Dzodzi Tsikata, interviewed in the documentary
The Witches of Gambaga

The belief of the childless that they may one day have a child can be matched by the dogmatic belief of those around them that their infertility is the sign of a curse, of some deep malevolence for which they are being punished. When this is the case, the stigmatization of those without offspring can become sinister and ritualized. Ghana is one such country where childlessness can lead to a woman being branded as a witch.

The capital of northern Ghana is Tamale. It is a predominantly Muslim town, proud of its rapid development, modern buildings and world-class sporting facilities. Just 150 kilometres to the north lies Gambaga, a former capital, now ravished by poverty and reduced to a rural settlement in the middle of an agricultural region. On the outskirts of the town is the witches' camp.[7]

There are four such camps in northern Ghana, two of which hold a handful of men (a survey in 1998 by the

Commission on Human Rights and Administrative Justice in Ghana stated that only thirteen male witches in total occupied the camps whereas there were over a thousand women). This is because, although men are often believed to be witches, it is thought that they are generally able to use their power more responsibly than women.

The camps are both a form of exile and a place of refuge. Until the late nineteenth century most women named as witches were executed, but when an imam intervened and saved a woman who was about to be put to death, the mosque became a place of sanctuary. Families built a motley collection of huts around the mosque, outwith the town itself, and banished the women to live in them. A quarrel between an imam and a local chief ended the witches' protection by the mosque and instead they were given over to the Chief of Gambaga, the Gambarana. Today's witches are still said to be under his shelter, prevented from practising their craft by the gods of Gambaga that he has conjured to watch over them.

The Gambarana protects the women but is also their jailer. They cannot leave the camp without his consent, even in the unlikely event that their families wish them to return home. They must pay for his protection, and if an outcast woman has no money then she pays by labouring for him. Thus the Gambarana encourages the belief that brings him a steady income and free labour while protecting the women from those who were once dearest to them.

The women who live in the camp tell stories of public beatings and humiliation before their arrival there. Childlessness is not the only reason they can be named a witch; mothers too can be abused and taunted, their homes may be looted and vandalized, their family refused any work in the area, eventually stripped of everything they possess. They come to the camp because others around them make it impossible for them to live anywhere else; once they are there, they are left alone.

But even when childlessness is not the explicit reason for exclusion, childless women recognize that they are more vulnerable and that having a son or daughter might have protected them from the accusations of witchcraft and their exile.

Childless women can be regarded either as witches or as people who have been cursed by a witch. Elderly childless women are thought to have magically traded the lives of children so that they themselves may live longer. These women are shunned by fellow villagers, jeered at when they venture from their houses, severely beaten if they attend any public events, lest they remain to enchant the children.[8] Both male and female fertility can also be offered up to the gods in exchange for wealth. This pledge can be reversed, but the cost is often greater than any wealth the childless person has, and the desperation to have children leaves them open to exploitation by medicine men and local healers. One Ghanaian man recounts: 'I have sacrificed several animals in an attempt to reverse a pledge I was told I made to the gods to be rich, yet the traditional healer is still demanding more, because he has seen that I am desperate to have a child.'[9]

Mary Osuma is sixty-five years old and lived in Gambaga for eight years. Born in Pontamale, she is the daughter of a Koranic scholar and has been married twice, but has not conceived a child in either marriage. She explained, 'My first husband was impotent. We lived in Accra. When I went back to Pontamale I explained the situation to my father and he decided to take me back from that man.' She married again and became a co-wife but 'There was no issue from my second marriage either. My husband already had a wife and two children.' Nevertheless she found happiness in the second union, her husband looked after her well and they didn't fight. But problems arose when others seemed to collude with the first wife against Mary. She left her husband and once again returned to her family, moving in with her brothers and their wives and children. She helped support the family financially, working as part of a cooperative called Amasachina, getting bank loans, using the money to trade.

The accusation that Mary was a witch came from within the cooperative. Ashitu, a young woman member, went to the chief of the village and said that she had dreamed that Mary and another woman, the deputy chairman of the cooperative, were chasing her. The village interpreted the dream as Mary and her co-accused wanting to kill Ashitu and banished them. Mary's co-accused had children and they took her to another village to settle there. Without children, Mary's only recourse was to her brother, who refused to shelter her in his house for fear of reprisals. Mary bore her brother no ill will: 'They would have killed me if I'd remained in Pontamale. They'd have killed my brother as well if he'd given me shelter. You see, we're strangers in the town. My father settled there. He wasn't a native of Pontamale.'

The accusation itself puzzled Mary; she had had no quarrel with Ashitu, and believed it was a conspiracy by the community, for which she could find no explanation beyond 'pure hatred'. She concluded, 'They wanted to get rid of me, and the other accused woman, even though Ashitu hadn't said we were trying to kill her; she'd simply said that she'd dreamt of us.'

Exile to Gambaga is preceded by a trial. Or a travesty of one. A ritual sacrifice shows whether or not the accused or the accuser is truthful. The Gambarana slits the throat of a chicken, which continues to skitter momentarily; the way it dies, whether with its wings facing down to the earth, or upwards to the sky, determines whether a woman is a witch or not. Mary's trial confirmed the suspicion of the community and she was condemned to exile in the witch's camp.

Yaba Badoe's powerful film *The Witches of Gambaga* shows another such trial. A chicken is bought and its throat slit by the Gambarana. It staggers off, flapping, panicking in its final throes. We wait. Wings facing upwards to the sky bring respite, while facing to the ground may bring decades within the witches' camp. In the film the ceremony is being performed for the second time in a woman's life. The first had found her to be a witch and condemned her to the camp; this second trial is because she longs to return to her family, who will pay the chief to allow her to do so. We wait together, the woman, her now reconciled family and the viewers. We watch as the bird dies with its wings spread upwards towards the sky, hear the clapping, feel the relief of the waiting circle, know that twenty years of exile are now ended.

The sacrifice of the bird has brought hope, the end of exclusion, For the childless woman it also removed responsibility for her state. The witch's camp was a place of exile, caught between community revilement and hopefulness, in the space where childlessness so often lives.

Those Who Believe: The Postcode Lottery

Faith is not limited to belief in the unknown; it's also the territory of medicine and science. But while the possibility of consolation or the fragile expectation of some miracle are open to anyone who has faith or might say a prayer, the more realistic option of in vitro fertilization is more expensive and therefore, as my husband and I discovered for ourselves, not available to everyone who might need or want it. Restrictions as to who qualifies for IVF in the UK include a range of factors, one of which is age. When I first went to a doctor with my symptoms of endometriosis, at the age of twenty-nine, I was well within the age limit for free IVF treatment. When I was thirty-six and my husband and I persisted together, we would still have qualified. But the years wasted in misdiagnosis or having my symptoms dismissed (one doctor sent me away after I'd passed out rather spectacularly in a supermarket, saying, 'Some women just have bad periods') meant that by the time IVF was posited as a solution, I was too old to qualify for it on the NHS in the area where we were living. Had I lived in the next borough, I would have been offered two cycles.

The organization Fertility Fairness was set up to highlight the inequitable provision of IVF and the long-term mental effects of infertility and to campaign for the right of all women in England to have access to the treatment recommended by the National Institute for Health and Care Excellence (NICE) in 2004.

NICE's clinical guidelines are clear. All eligible women aged under forty should be entitled to three full cycles of IVF. Investigations conducted by Fertility Fairness show that in 2015 only 18 per cent of Clinical Commissioning Groups (CCGs) provided three such cycles, and more than half provided only one. Where this reduced treatment was on offer, it did not conform to NICE's definition of a cycle, so women are in effect having a partial cycle of IVF that greatly restricts their chances of falling pregnant.

It's a situation that is getting worse, not better. Since I started researching this book, the number of cycles available and the number of CCGs offering any IVF is steadily decreasing. Statistics bear it out: Fertility Fairness research shows that between 2013 and 2015 the CCGs offering three cycles decreased from 24 per cent to 18 per cent, and by 2017 that figure had dropped again to just 12 per cent.[10]

Additionally, the eligibility criteria for any treatment vary greatly depending on where you live. Age can be one – 6 per cent of CCGs restrict fertility treatment to women under thirty-five, despite the recommendations that all women should be eligible for one complete cycle up to the age of forty-two; the time spent trying to conceive can be another criterion, even when there is an identified medical cause of infertility.

Scotland and Wales are more equitable, in that they offer all eligible women under forty three cycles of treatment. In England the division is almost a north-south divide: northern CCGs generally offer far more cycles than those in the south-east, but the differences even within a city like London are astonishing. Camden alone of the London CCGs offers three full cycles of IVF. Islington offer two, Barnet offer one and so on. Your CCG is determined by the location of your doctor's surgery, not your home, so by finding a GP practice in a better catchment that will accept patients from your postcode, you can move the odds just a little bit in your favour.[11]

Melanie and her husband Tom are childless and wish they were not. When they were trying to get pregnant, Primary Care Trusts administered IVF treatment rather than CCGs, but the differences were just as pronounced.[12] Melanie is a cheerful woman, now in her forties, with the kind of wide smile that includes you in its happiness. But her demeanour has come about through acceptance, not by resolution of her situation. They live on a council estate, in an immaculate terraced house that reminds me of my mother's – the kind of place we used to say was so clean you could eat your meal off the floor. There are baby pictures on the sideboard, of a niece and a goddaughter, and a wedding portrait where Melanie's unchanged smile brings all the clichés of a bride being radiant to mind.

Women are born with a set number of eggs; these eggs deplete as you age, bleed out of you each month. But their quantity can also be diminished by chemotherapy, which was what happened to Melanie. In her twenties, she was successfully treated for cancer with a combination of radiotherapy and chemotherapy. The memory of the physical effects of the chemo – the vomiting, the weakness – still causes a cloud to come across her face when she speaks of them, but it was the invisible legacy that caught up with her later. Melanie still had eggs in her mid-thirties, when she and Tom first tried to have a child, but she didn't have as many as most women of her age. Melanie answers a question I would never ask but that countless people before me presumably have: 'We would probably have had babies even younger, but I had to take a break from taking the tamoxifen first.' After six months of trying unsuccessfully, they went to have a consultation about IVF.

Some of Melanie's eggs had been gathered and frozen before her cancer treatment, so she assumed that she would be able to begin treatment with her frozen eggs. But no. The steroids she had taken during treatment had led to weight gain and she was now outside of the body mass index set by her health authority. First she had to diet. After four months Melanie was the correct weight for treatment. But by then she was thirty-nine and in her postcode the cut-off for IVF on the NHS was thirty-eight, not forty, as it was in many others.

There was a possibility of 'exceptional funding', but Melanie's gynaecologist, a woman she describes as completely sympathetic and supportive, explained that it might take up to two years to be approved. More time off tamoxifen was also a risk. 'We sold our flat and moved in with my mum,' Melanie told me, and paid for private IVF treatment. 'This is actually her house. Tom and I have the two rooms upstairs. We're saving to see if we can get a place of our own again, but it just gets more and more difficult.' The IVF didn't work. Tom and Melanie went through five cycles using the money left after paying off the mortgage on their flat. 'Now we're homeless and childless, but I still have Tom and Mum's been great.' Melanie smiled. 'Not sure I would have coped if I had been like so many of the other women I see in my support group, whose husbands have all left them.'

Melanie's group is not atypical. A Danish study of 47,500 women found that those who didn't have a child after treatment were three times more likely to divorce or separate from their partner than those who were successful.[13]

'Once we have enough to get a two-bed place, we've decided to adopt. At the moment we're not eligible, because we don't have a home at all, but Tom's doing lots of overtime and we'll get there. And, looking on the bright side, my cancer has never come back. It might have taken away so many possibilities for my life, but it's also changed my outlook completely. I know adoption isn't for everyone, and of course it's an entirely different thing from having my own baby, but it's what we want for us, now. Our new hope, if you like.'

English politicians may put access to fertility treatment low on their agenda because it's not a vote winner and public opinion is divided about whether it should be available at all, and, if so, to whom. Yet the original NICE recommendations were clear; this isn't a question of changing a medical decision or policy, but of ensuring that those guidelines are applied consistently and fairly. Arguments based on cost are also much less straightforward when you consider that the World Health Organization classifies infertility as a disease and that the cost of leaving it untreated leads to depression, stress and 'other serious long-term health costs', all of which will be treated out of the NHS budget.

But disparity of access isn't the only issue to blight the hope offered by IVF in Britain. Just as the religiously devout may be exploited in their desperation, so too may the people, mainly women, who turn to the fertility industry. Lord Robert Winston, Emeritus Professor of Fertility Studies at Imperial College, frequently criticizes prevalent bad practice as well as highlighting the inadequacy of the Human Fertilization and Embryology Authority (HFEA), the government's regulatory body, in dealing with it.

The practice of egg sharing is promoted as a means by

which a woman who cannot afford IVF, and is ineligible for help on the NHS, can access treatment. The woman has her ovaries stimulated by drugs so that she produces eggs. One or two of these eggs will be put into her own womb, while the others will go to another patient who does not have eggs of her own. This second woman will pay for both her own IVF and that of the egg donor. The problem arises when there are surplus eggs. As Professor Winston explains: 'This means that, for the clinics, persuading women to donate their eggs can be extremely lucrative. It also means that clinics have an incentive to maximise the chance of getting as many eggs as possible.'[14]

Unscrupulous clinics may stimulate a woman more than is necessary to produce more eggs, despite the fact that the eggs obtained may be of poorer quality or the process may be injurious to her health. While a donor's treatment may be unsuccessful, her eggs may result in children for someone else. On reaching adulthood, this child or these children would then by law have the right to know who their genetic mother is. So it is possible that years later, a childless, grieving woman, whose own treatment has failed, could be traced and visited by a child she didn't know existed.[15] Yet clinics are dismissive of patients' concerns.

Professor Winston also attacks many of the claims about the success of egg freezing. Various London clinics offering the service give high success rates for their patients. A newspaper investigation reports a consultant telling a woman her chance of pregnancy is 65 per cent, yet figures from the HFEA suggest a live birth rate of around 1.5 per cent is more likely.[16] Professor Winston argues, 'Most lay people would assume that, if they attend this clinic, they are close to being guaranteed a pregnancy. This seems very misleading and the HFEA should step in.'[17]

The lack of action by the HFEA means that women are at risk of exploitation from avaricious, profit-motivated clinics. The very women who may have doubted the honesty or efficacy of faith-based healing find that their childlessness is also a lure for a different kind of corruption, one that is cloaked in the respectability of medicine.

Those Who Believe in Chance

All you have to do is walk along the Las Vegas Strip to feel the atmosphere of expectation. Neon signs proclaim that a millionaire is being made this very minute, while quiet observation of the tattered men and women who mushroom on the streets early in the morning and last thing at night tells you that far more people are losing everything they have in search of that very possibility. Rainbow Boulevard runs parallel to the Strip. On its southern stretch, at the point where, a few blocks east, the pyramid of the Luxor hotel shines a pure white light in which a thousand moths swirl and flutter, there is an anonymous pale pink and red building that houses the Sher Institute. There are no lottery signs or gambling adverts, but the people who go there take a chance in any case. It's a fertility clinic, renowned for its high success rate and the ebullient personality of its South African celebrity specialist, Dr Geoffrey Sher.

Only fifteen states have passed laws that make it compulsory for health insurers to include infertility treatment in their plans. In the others, such as Nevada, it's often excluded or only partially covered, but this clinic does offer a plan where would-be parents can pay off the total amount in monthly instalments Even then, the cost, which is well out of the reach of many, only offers a chance. Nurse Linda Vignapiano, the clinical director of Sher, describes a scenario where you take twenty thousand dollars to a car lot to buy a car. You hand over your money, but you only have a fifty-fifty chance of then getting any keys. 'Would you even gamble on that?' she asks.

The Sher Institute, far more controversially, until recently ran a yearly competition where infertile women and couples could compete for a single free cycle of IVF. The contest, based on social-media, was called 'I Believe', as is the theme song for the institute, an easy-listening acoustic number sung by a good-looking couple which includes lines like:

I believe that there's a change around the corner
And in a world that's out of order I still have time.[18]

It sounds exactly like a charismatic Christian song, carefully designed to stay in your memory, uplifting, but also emotionally manipulative. It is very good at what it does. I listen and feel by turns cross that I am beguiled, but also, for the first time in years, a little sad that we really did run out of time.

The contestants had to make a video of themselves, telling their journey, and post it online. The viewers then voted for their favourites and a shortlist was made. From the shortlist just one winner was chosen by a panel of fertility experts and patients. A documentary, *Vegas Baby* (2016), looked at some of the hopeful entrants from 2013 and interviewed the staff at the clinic. Linda Vignapiano explained why she refused to have anything to do with the competition: 'I don't like pitting these people against each other.'

Keiko Zoll, editor of *The Infertility Voice*, was invited to be a judge and refused: 'It's the one sector of the entire health spectrum where it seems entirely normal to have a raffle or a contest. It's disturbing.' But Dr Sher defended the practice: 'It's a hardship for the average American to afford IVF and for many it's impossible. For those that say there shouldn't be a contest, I agree. There should be insurance.' The contest was obviously excellent for the clinic's finances and Sher was adamant that that's what medicine is partly about: 'People think of medicine as a calling. It is a calling, but it is also a business.' Sher stressed that there were two objectives: the first was to raise awareness and give the possibility of pregnancy to a couple who couldn't afford it; the second was to build his brand. The first objective was 'altruistic and that's great, but it's not how the world works'.

The posted homemade films were difficult to watch; even the excerpts in the documentary were upsetting. The psychologist Carl Rogers argues that humans have a natural potential to grow positively which is stunted by the judgement of others.[19] These videos were online, on YouTube, on Facebook, for everyone to see, watch, comment on and judge. Those who did not win might once again feel they were undeserving of a child. It was not the upturned wing of a chicken, but it was the arbitrary personal judgement of whoever happened to be looking at their story at the time of the voting.

But then, of course, one couple might have their life transformed. The system is unfair. It is a different kind of inequity from in the UK, but the net result is the same: if

you have money and are infertile, you can at least try to do
something about it; if you don't, there are different kinds of
lotteries you can enter to gain that possibility.

Infertility is still shrouded in the kind of embarrassment
usually reserved for incontinence. A recent survey by
Infertility UK showed that a third of their 500 respondents
were embarrassed by their inability to have a child.[20] Many of
the 'I Believe' competitors felt they were 'outing themselves'
about their condition, something they had previously only
shared with family and close friends. One of the competitors
described being infertile as 'one of the most humiliating
things you can experience'. In some cases secrecy about the
decision to enter the contest was professionally necessary.
One of the contestants was the manager of a Catholic
television station – and even the judging panel wondered
if his publicly posted film to win medical treatment that
the Roman Catholic church disapproves of could lead to
his dismissal. Yet he and his wife took the chance. In their
film they were surrounded by family; they spoke of the
importance of family in the Mexican culture, their repeated
failure, the money they had lost chasing their hope, their
belief that they could and would have a baby, one day.

Other contestants, Brian and Ann Johnson, from Green
Bay, Wisconsin, spoke of the mortgage they took out to pay
for IVF, the joy when two eggs took, then the heartbreak
of the stillbirth of one baby followed by the twin's death
three weeks later in a premature birth. They tried adoption
next, but after just a year the child they were fostering was
reclaimed by the birth mother. Ann has endometriosis and
polycystic ovary syndrome and they had been trying for
seven years. Brian confessed to the camera that he has to

fight the 'urge to say, I'm done, I want to move on', because the tragedy piled up between them seems too immense to live with. Ann looked at him when he said that and it was clear she was terrified as well as sad.

Watching the film, despite all of my misgivings, I found that I was helplessly rooting for Brian and Ann. In part it was illness-empathy, I think. Not all of the contestants had medical reasons for their childlessness. But it was also sadness for their misfortunes, one on top of the other. I believed they deserved a bit of luck. In a Vegas clinic, what could be more fitting? They won the contest. Their story appealed to the public, as it had to me, so they were shortlisted, and then, at the next stage, selected by the judges, who also factored in the likely success of the procedure. In the end they had their baby. Their mortgage was foreclosed and they had to rent a smaller house, but they were both ecstatic. For Brian the contest was a means: 'This is what we had to do to get our family.'

A Short Note on the Naming of Things

On a plane heading for the United States, I flick through the on-screen entertainment list and settle on a film called *By the Sea*. Angelina Jolie plays the leading female character and I find her loveliness astonishing, even in a world where we are constantly assailed by promoted and manufactured beauty. I know nothing about the content of the film. I choose to watch it simply because I like Jolie.

But then unexpectedly, as it unfolds before me, I see it is about the effects of childlessness, and at one point when the male protagonist, played by Brad Pitt, hurls the word 'barren' at his wife, I find myself flinching in my tightly packed, airless world. My husband is beside me, oblivious to the high-ceilinged Mediterranean room my imagination has inhabited, caught instead in some grim battle fought by grotesque creatures on the small screen pulled out in front of him. I squeeze his arm. He smiles at me. I feel soothed. But the word 'barren' lingers in my head like the sting of a slap.

Sticks and stones
Can break my bones
But words can never harm me.

It's true enough. I have a fleeting image of a woman beaten by her neighbours, even her family, with sticks, with fists, cast out of her home and village. I know that I am fortunate. But oh, how I hate this word. I am thankful I have never been called it in anger. It seems to be everything I am not. I hope it is everything I am not. It's true my body could not sustain a child, but my hair and my nails grow, my skin flakes and dies and renews itself and I hope my mind develops. I have lived in a desert and travelled across Death Valley. While they are landscapes that I love, I should hate to consider myself represented by them. To think of it, even Death Valley is not barren; far from it. One spring my husband and I drove across those plains and were moved by the proliferation of flowers – multitudinous, kaleidoscopic in their shapes and colours. We felt as if we had been gifted to see them in one of the short, rare times that they blossom. But a woman labelled as barren is denied even that possibility, that moment of transformation.

The idiomatic links between the landscape and child-bearing are international and there seem to be no exceptions, but the cultural unacceptability in many societies of a woman who does not have children, as opposed to a man who does not, is a different thing altogether.

I start to collect the words for 'childless', for 'infertile', for *barren*, in other languages. In Greek a landscape which is not fertile and men and women who cannot have children are στείρος/στείρα (*stiros/stira*), but in the Cypriot countryside the far more derogatory term μαρμάρα (*marmara*), literally a sheep or goat that cannot have young, is used only for women. In Sinhala ඩෙ (*vanda*) means, literally, unable to produce and generally refers to trees in an orchard. However, when used to describe a woman, it is offensive and rude. In Polish the gender distinction is even more etched into the language.

The terms for a person who is childless are *bezdzietna* (for a woman) and *bezdzietny* (for a man). When applied to a woman, this is often accompanied by another word meaning angry and unfulfilled, to give *bezdzietna jezda*. It's a term often used to describe a childless woman, even in a context where it is irrelevant whether she is a parent or not, and has only negative connotations, but there is no equivalent in use for childless men. In Italian the word *zitella* is derogatory in the extreme and means an unmarried, childless woman, but there is no equivalent for men. In rural Bangladesh there are eighteen different words used almost exclusively for women who cannot have children, from *poramukhi*, 'burnt face' – someone who has a face that burns and spoils other people's happiness – to *olokhkhi*, 'poor, miserable'.[1]

But to say that it is always thus, that the negative terms are either female or neutral, would be to neglect other languages, those from a few cultures where a childless man may carry the same shame as a woman and whose vernacular conveys this. There are parts of rural India where fertility is as highly valued for men as it is for women, and men who cannot impregnate their wives may be barred from social events and celebrations and mockingly called *kliba* or *napunska*, 'a sexually dysfunctional non-man'.[2] In Ghana the taunts are more explicit still, and a man can be derided as *lankpolosoba*, 'a man with rotten testes', or *yokuusoba*, 'a man with a dead penis'.[3]

For me, this gathering of words becomes almost a talismanic thing, as if by their number, their universality, and then by their reduction to a collection on a page, I might diffuse their power to wound.

They should form a collection of aridity, made infertile

themselves, incapable of breeding hurt or shame, reduced
to black marks on a page, some far less familiar than others,
curious in their strangeness. Pinned objects, worthy of
investigation. Curios. Objects of scientific consideration. But
it is a futile wish; I find that I am only able to look at them
dispassionately when I do not think too much at all, when I
do not imagine a young woman in Bangladesh, hiding her
face in her hands, or in a scorched red strip of cloth, because
she too has begun to wonder if it brings ill will to those who
look on it.

3

Those Who Were Denied

While the British government stealthily and inconsistently decides who may or may not be given the chance to have a child through IVF, other political organizations elsewhere did not care about such subtleties. Eugenic sterilization is most often associated with the Nazi Party during the Second World War, but by the late twentieth century it had become apparent that numerous societies implemented involuntary sterilization programmes until as recently as the 1980s. These countries included Austria, Denmark, Switzerland, Sweden and Canada. News reports in the 1990s revealed that 60,000 people, predominantly women, were sterilized in Sweden between 1935 and 1976 in one such programme, established by the Institute for Racial Biology.[1]

Following on from the international revelations, two Canadian scholars, D. C. Park and J. Radford, looked into the case files of the Eugenics Board of Alberta. The implementation of forcible sterilization for those deemed 'mentally deficient' was well attested in North America. In 1928 the Sexual Sterilization Act was passed in Alberta after a campaign and intense pressure from the United Farm Women's Association, who argued that their own farm stock had been greatly improved by following eugenic principles.

Originally the procedure was meant to require consent, but in practice this meant that victims had to agree or were threatened with permanent incarceration and punishment. By 1937 even the pretence of patient collusion ended and the existing Sterilization Act was strengthened so that consent was no longer required from anyone regarded as mentally deficient, and it remained so until 1972. What was unusual about Alberta was that, unlike elsewhere in North America, the number of operations on the 'mentally handicapped' reached its peak in the 1950s and 1960s, when they were 'couched under the rubric of liberalism and humanitarianism'.[2]

Unlike the numerous papers examining the legislation or medical practice of the act, Park and Radford consider individual cases by looking at the files kept by officialdom. It's a grim, dispassionate account, presenting the words of the state that enforced the dictate rather than anything of the personal feelings or stories of the victims. But it does show the reasons submitted for each case and gives a glimpse of the 'rationales of the asylum'. And therein lies the irony, embedded in a phrase, because within those 'institutes of madness' an insane logic prevailed. Far more women than men were operated on. Men would have either a vasectomy or, occasionally, have both testicles removed. With women, the process involved the surgical removal of a fallopian tube or, in the most drastic cases, the ovaries.

The precise justification for such procedures varied and present a chilling, almost surreal list:

Behavioural difficulties (abnormal sexual behaviour, destructive and criminal tendencies)

Deprivation of family support (parental death, spousal
abandonment, illegitimate offspring, referral to a social
welfare agency)
Impoverished family environment
Precondition to institutional release
Parental request[3]

Individual descriptions give further insight. A seventeen-
year-old woman was sterilized in 1946 because she was
'rather bossy and bad tempered in her own home', liked
to go out alone and freely chatted to people she met, and
had additionally been sexually assaulted three years earlier.[4]
A fifteen-year-old girl was operated on because the board
reported that her family was dependent on the state and
had been on relief and Mother's Allowance for years.[5] Being
abandoned by her parents and showing a 'lively interest in
the opposite sex' were the grounds for a sixteen-year-old
to lose the possibility of ever having a child of her own. In
1951, an illegitimate girl, just fourteen, described as being
of 'Indian blood', was sterilized after being diagnosed as
'mentally defective'. She had been sexually assaulted six
times by her stepfather. The cases of male sterilization,
while far fewer in number, are no less moving. A 'friendly,
co-operative' twenty-five-year-old man, who 'was fond of
animals' and 'demonstrated no interest in the opposite sex',
was operated on because both his parents had died and the
state was unable to appoint a guardian.[6]

But what became of men and women such as these? How
did they manage to negotiate a life that was not of their own
making? In one case at least there was a good outcome.

On 25 January 1996 Leilani Muir won a landmark court

case against the Alberta government. In the Canadian Film Board documentary *The Sterilization of Leilani Muir*, she is referred to as 'a symbol of everybody else who was touched by that act', and her story, because of its detail, profile and publicity, as well as her continuing campaign to raise awareness for other victims, represents a window of understanding of the suffering that was caused.

Leilani was raised in an abusive house. Often hungry, she took to stealing sandwiches from other children's lunch boxes; when teachers realized the reason, they brought food in for her themselves. But the family moved often; Leilani recounts how any visit to question her parental care would mean another farmhouse in a different area. The houses were remote, without neighbours, and Leilani was kept out of sight, unwanted by a mother who openly said she had never wished for a daughter. Even before she was eleven years old, she was admitted to a provincial training school; her mother no longer wished to have her at home and, according to Leilani, lied so that she might be admitted.

Within four months, she was given an IQ test, used by the school to measure mental competency, and her score of sixty-four left her branded as a 'moron'. Her confinement there would last for a decade but, after only four years, under the pretext of undergoing an appendectomy, her fallopian tube was removed. It wasn't until she was released and married for the first time that Leilani knew what had been done to her; the examining doctor told her that her insides looked as if she had been 'through a slaughterhouse'.[7] The operation was not reversible – there just wasn't enough tubal length for reconstruction.

When I heard this, I had an image of doctors trying to

catch onto tissue, to somehow elongate the remains and make them viable again, but futilely as it slipped between their hopeful fingers, too thin and fragile to hold. It was an image that was familiar and seemed to represent so much of childlessness: the body's inability to hold and nurture a life within it, because its parts were damaged, deformed or broken, whether by illness or human agency.

Leilani was awarded three quarters of a million dollars but, in reply to a journalist's question, she said that it could not compensate her for what she had lost and would continue to miss for as long as she lived. How could there be a price on the life of a child?

Those Who Were Denied: Racially Motivated Sterilization

In 1991 I was working with groups of Roma from Yugoslavia (as it was then) who had settled in the UK. I had been awarded a grant and I travelled from Sheffield, where I had my first academic position, to London on alternate weekends, usually staying with one of my closest friends and his flatmates on a battered couch in their shared living room in Kilburn. It was a strange mode of existence. I owned a small flat in Sheffield, had new lecture courses to prepare, and, even if I had been able to find more time for going out, I didn't really know anyone there. In contrast, my weekends were crammed and sleepless, taken up with as many meetings with my research subjects as I could arrange and socializing with university friends. Despite the fact that I had a steady income, my mode of living was little different to

when I was a student. I was in my mid-twenties. I had every
intention that one day I would have children, preferably
soon – thirty seemed like the perfect age to me – but I had no
real commitment to anyone or any place. Of all my friends,
Michael, whose couch was my weekend bed, was the one
who was most determined to have children. When we spoke
about it, the question mark was always about when we might
meet the right person, and never, ever, about whether or not
we might be physically able to.

I was studying the Romany language and was interested
in a particular aspect of the culture that had not been
much written about. The Kalderesh are a subgroup of the
Romany people and *marimei* traditions and hygiene taboos
are strict behavioural codes observed within many Kalderesh
households. *Marimei* seemed to highlight the importance of
fecundity to the community, a fact that was secondary to my
research but which now, when I play the old tape recordings on a still-functioning cassette recorder that I had as a
university student, seems far more urgent and interesting
than my clinical observations of the time. Listening back, I
was reminded of Paul Kalanithi's observation in his memoir
When Breath Becomes Air: 'Science may provide the most
useful way to organize empirical, reproducible data, but its
power to do so is predicated on its inability to grasp the most
central aspects of human life: hope, fear, love, hate, beauty,
envy, honour, weakness, striving, suffering, virtue.'[8]

The code of *marimei* dictates what is allowed or forbidden,
is literally clean or unclean, within a family group. Women
or girls who are too young to menstruate, or are unmarried
(marriage is generally at a very young age), are *sholhi* or *shebari*.
They are assumed to be virginal, and therefore incapable of

causing pollution in the ways that a married, widowed or divorced woman can. These young women often enjoyed a degree of freedom of movement within the home as well as an exemption from the dress code that was imposed on the other women in the house. However, part of a girl's up-bringing is to learn how she must conduct herself once she becomes a *boori*, a married woman; most importantly she has to learn how to avoid contaminating or polluting those around her in the household. An action that breaches these rules of cleanliness and avoidance, or an object that has become tainted in this way, is said to be *marimei*.[9]

What was distinct about the Yugoslavian families was that, unlike in English gypsy communities, it was not illicit sex that made the women unclean and therefore capable of pollution, but any sex at all.[10] Offspring perform a vital role in allowing the *boori* to interact with her family by creating a barrier between her polluted state and the world around her. Without offspring, many simple tasks become difficult or even impossible in some stricter homes, thus further isolating the woman even within her own family.

Katerina was from Kosovo and lived in Hammersmith. She lived with her husband's parents and Sara, her younger sister-in-law, in a large terraced house. Even though she had been married for six years, there were no children. Later in our friendship, Katerina admitted that, while she didn't want to hold Sara back from the joys of marriage, she dreaded the day that she would leave the house and not be there to act as her intermediary. I asked her what she meant and she gestured to the long dark skirt that all the married Kalderesh women wore. 'This skirt, the very clothes I wear, are all *marimei*. If I brush against a man other than my husband, I can make him poisoned too. If my husband is watching a man on the television, I cannot walk between him and the TV set but must go all around the room, even if I am carrying many things. It is not until I have my own daughters that they will be able to help me.'[11]

Katerina was insistent that it was only a matter of time before 'the dam would break' and she would have 'one child, then many, many children', and indeed over the three years of our meetings, she gave birth to a healthy boy. But through my friendship with Katerina I met another Roma woman, younger and apparently single, from what was then the Slovakian region of Czechoslovakia. Her name was Rosa.[12] She was twenty-four and she would never have children because, without her knowledge, the government had stripped her of that right.

It took time to learn her story. My knowledge of the language was imperfect, Katerina had to translate for me, and decades of discrimination have made many Roma understandably wary of prying *gaje* (non-Roma) and their questions. I was only slightly older and her situation was barely comprehensible to me. I sympathized but could not empathize, because her story seemed embedded within the landscape and culture that she had grown up in. My world was late-night clubs, not enough sleep and ill-advised encounters. These were things that I believed would all be abandoned when children came, and in no way precluded the domesticity I imagined before me. Rosa's landscape had written her fate, her childlessness, indelibly and legibly on her body, whereas I had not yet learned to read the marks on mine, although they were there, carrying messages I was unable to decipher.

When she was sixteen, Rosa was raped by a *gaje*. Her family and other Roma had been moved from the village where they had lived all their lives and were travelling towards the city, where they thought there might be work and a better chance of avoiding discrimination. They spent the nights of their two-day journey in makeshift tents. 'I couldn't sleep,' Rosa told Katerina, who interpreted for me. 'I know what I did was wrong and that in so many ways this is all my own fault. But I went for a walk, just a short walk, to get away from everyone – the babies and my mother's sadness and my father telling me that I would have to marry soon. I left the safety of my family and he grabbed me and took me. I bled a lot afterwards. I was so ashamed and afraid anyone would know that I had gone out on my own like that, I told my sister I had my period and wore a towel for the bleeding. It hurt. I knew there was blood when you lost your virginity because we often display the blood after the first night.' Katerina nodded as she translated this. 'But I hadn't expected this.'

When Rosa found she was pregnant, she confessed what had happened to her mother, who took her to the hospital nearest to the town where they had temporarily settled with her father's cousins. Rosa's father refused to speak to her, but her mother supported her. 'She was kind and I hadn't expected it. It made me feel silly for not having gone to her in the first place. My mum said Dad would be better once we'd got rid of the child, and I knew she was right. In any case, it made me feel dirty, like I was carrying the memory of that man inside me. I was happier than I had been since it happened when they told me that I was in time for the operation.'[13]

Rosa signed a form agreeing to an abortion. She could write her name, but her mother, who was illiterate, had to countersign with an X. Neither of them could read the long document, but it was presented as their agreement to the termination.

Rosa remembers being given an injection and waking up in pain. But within a few days she had recovered and the whole extended family moved again, this time to Lunik IX, the infamous Roma slum in the western part of Kosice. Her father once again acknowledged her, and a wedding was arranged with Marco, the son of one of the families who had travelled with them. 'I liked him and he had an elder brother, Irek, in London, who promised to help us get out of Lunik.'

Rosa hated the slum. In the 2012 documentary *Lunik IX*, we can see streets filled with garbage, rubble strewn in front rooms where a wall has partially collapsed, residents scavenging at the landfill area in front of the vast blocks for pieces of wood or old furniture to burn because there is no gas or electricity. Even water is only available for an hour at a time between morning and afternoon, and so family members shuttle between their homes and outdoor taps laden with plastic containers, in order to be able to stay clean or cook their food.

For most of the Roma, it was seen as a place of no possible escape, yet, with her marriage, Rosa did just that. Her brother-in-law helped Marco and Rosa to find their way through the complicated miasma of British immigration; Marco took a job at a second-hand-car garage, and they stayed in Irek's terraced house, living in two rooms and a bathroom. 'I was happy, but then the months and years passed and I didn't have children and it was clear he was disappointed in me.'

Rosa went to a London hospital, only to be told that she had been sterilized and wouldn't be able to have a child. The horror of the discovery brought understanding. It was not her fault. Marco divorced her. 'But he's a kind man,' she told us. 'He didn't send me back to Slovakia to my family but let me move in with other relations of his and work for them. I don't have a bad life. But I could have had a lovely one, with children. I so wanted to have a baby of my own.' My recording ends on that line. At the time, I listened carefully to the original Kalderesh, trying to pick out when, elicited by me, Rosa used the terms *sholhi* and *boori* to refer to herself, and of course it was before and after the sexual attack, although she used *sholhi* once again when she spoke about her wedding, which I found touching. Years later, I can't understand any of the Romani language and I struggle to pick out even my familiar research terms. I find now that it's Katerina's interpreting that moves me – the way I hear in her voice her sympathy for her friend's pain, and her struggle to put it aside so she can give me as accurate an account as possible.

Rosa's case was not unique. The sterilization of the Roma in Slovakia became an international scandal. Like the Canadian cases, the justification for many of the sterilizations was partly entrenched in a belief that the white immigrant settlers were superior, and that this superiority had to be protected and nurtured by preventing too much dilution. But in the case of the Roma, the justification lay in racist assumptions, not criteria of mental competency. Furthermore there was (and still is) a feeling across swathes of Europe that the Roma population were lazy, living off the state, and so represented an economic burden that had to be limited in any way feasible. The Communist regime in Czechoslovakia had a policy of assimilating the Roma, which included curbing their traditionally high fertility rates, by force if necessary, but this officially ended with the collapse of the regime in 1990. However, a number of doctors continued the practice. It was systemic but unacknowledged. A Czech health ministry advisory committee finally concluded only that 'procedural mistakes have been made in a number of cases',[14] but the Czech embassy in London refused to acknowledge that the sterilizations had been part of a national policy targeting an ethnic group.

Barbara Bukovska, a lawyer and human-rights activist, founded the Center for Civil and Human Rights in Slovakia in an attempt to bring the treatment of Roma to international attention. In a 2003 documentary, *The Sterilization of Roma Women*, she comments that the prevailing local fear is that the Roma are going to outnumber the Slovaks and that such measures are justified because they are protecting society. In the film, staff at Presov Hospital, often named in connection with the practice, openly refer to the Roma as a 'degenerate race' given to 'sexual relations between brother and sister, father and daughter, mother and son'. Jud Nirenberg, a representative from the Carpathian Foundation NGO, summarizes the prevalent Slovak attitude as a belief that the Roma lack basic human characteristics.[15]

Bukovska compiled a report of her findings in 2003: *Body and Soul: Forced Sterilization and Other Assaults on Roma Reproductive Freedom in Slovakia*. It concluded that of 200 Roma women interviewed from eastern Slovakia, at least

110 had been coerced or forced into sterilization. Slovakia was due to become a full member of the European Union in 2004 and the government retaliated by prosecuting Bukovska. The report was backed by Amnesty International and the Human Rights Commissioner of the Council of Europe,[16] yet the courts prevaricated. Slovakia joined the EU. The women's cases did not progress, despite constant lobbying by the Center for Civil and Human Rights. Then, in 2009, Bukovska won the right for the forcibly sterilized women to access their medical documents and the evidence could no longer be withheld. Several cases were won in the European Court of Human Rights, which acknowledged the forcible sterilization of the Roma women and found this in contravention of Article 3 (prohibition of inhuman or degrading treatment) and Article 8 (right to respect for private and family life) of the European Convention. On 13 November 2012 the European Court of Human Rights finally awarded damages to two Roma women who had been sterilized without their knowledge in Slovakia, on the grounds that the operation constituted inhuman and degrading treatment. However, the judges refused to rule on the women's claim that the procedure had been racially motivated, a ruling that was received with dismay by Roma activists and some human rights lawyers.[17]

Those Who Were Denied: So Many Voices

The Quipu Project was created in conjunction with Amnesty International to tell the story of the mutilation of the indigenous women of the Peruvian Andes. Their website does not just give a platform to their accounts but also opens lines of communication across the world. The project began by giving women in many remote Andean villages mobile phones and a free number to call, inviting them to share their stories. These phones were connected to the internet, recordings of the women's testimonies were transcribed and translated into Quechua, Spanish and English and then uploaded into an archive which can be listened to anywhere in the world that has an internet connection. Listeners can leave a message for the women too – to record their emotions, their feeling of solidarity and admiration, to tell them we have listened, we have heard.

Khipu is the word for 'knot' in Quechua. A *quipu* consisted of a group of coloured threads – anything from a handful to two thousand – whose knots and colours were used to communicate and record information in the Andes. The oldest *quipu* dates from the first millennium AD and today there is still ritual significance attached to these historical objects within Andean communities. They give the Quipu Project its name, but the thin threads that appear on the website represent the virtual telephone lines reaching from Andean villages out across the world.[18]

During the 1990s, 272,000 women and 22,000 men were sterilized in Peru, mostly without consent, often without awareness of what was being done to them. The circumstances of each of the women were different. One woman was prevented from registering her one-month-old daughter and getting her birth certificate unless she consented to sterilization; another went to give birth and left sterilized and without a baby; others were threatened with having food or support withdrawn if they did not have the procedure.[19]

News of the atrocities filtered through to the international media gradually. Then, in 1999, the documentary *Secret Sterilization* brought pictures and testimony from rural Peru to a wider audience. 'The Thread' the presenter tells us, is the word the women use for a hysterectomy.[20] It is an image that presages the threads of the Quipu Project; I imagine them not only as fragile lines of communication but as a physical violation, a bloody trail leading to each of the women.

In Huancavelica, one of the poorest rural areas, a native woman called Madalena Reginaldo is interviewed. She testifies to the operation, but also to the horrific experience of waking up during her hysterectomy and her pain being disregarded by the medical team around her. 'I felt pain,' Madalena says. 'They were cutting into me and I wanted to get up. I said, doctor, it's hurting, and he just told me the anaesthetic wasn't working.'

Many of these women are not childless and the information is incomplete, so I have no idea which women have children now. What is sure is that the state has denied them the possibility of having more in the future, by performing either a hysterectomy or a tubal ligation, so if they are or become childless, that is how they will remain. The documentary I watched was filmed in the 1990s, yet only in November 2015 did the Peruvian government acknowledge that its citizens' rights had been violated, declaring 'of national interest the priority attention of victims of forced sterilization produced between 1995 and 2001.'[21]

I hear incomprehensible voices, read translated words. Mostly they tell of physical pain, a few include the phrase 'I live alone'. The women are anonymous, and it is impossible to know why they are alone. Do they have husbands?

Children? One woman tells of physical pain then adds, 'Our husbands tell us we are nothing.' Another speaker, like many others, says that since she was sterilized she can no longer lift anything, is not able to do the work she needs to do just to live in her rural community. She too lives alone. With the loss of fertility, the women have lost not only the value that fertility brings in their culture and their community but the physical ability to contribute to the group. The operations were often performed in unhygienic environments by barely trained staff. There was no post-operative care, no transport to take the women home, so, still raw from the operation, in some cases they would walk miles and miles just to get back to their village.

The multitudinous accounts are powerful. Many are similar. But their alikeness does not diminish them; it makes them stronger, truer. They are a chorus of condemnation, each voice an integral part of the whole. Every woman is unique and must be acknowledged. I am unquestionably outside of my remit; I am listening to mothers, who call themselves such, and who mourn unborn children as well as the physical attributes of a healthy body. I listen anyway and I write. I cannot bring myself to click the 'next thread' icon every time a woman mentions that she has a son or a daughter, or was only sterilized when they took her in ostensibly to help her with the birth of a child.

Those Who were Denied: Cultural Practice

Female genital mutilation (FGM) is a cultural practice in many, generally patriarchal societies. Globally there are over 200 million cases, in more than thirty countries, where it is usually performed on young girls, regarded as a way to mark the rite of passage into womanhood. The phrase female genital mutilation actually relates to four different procedures, all of which involve 'partial or total removal of the female genitalia without medical reasons'. The World Health Organization classifies these four as:

1. Partial or total removal of the clitoris and or prepuce
2. Partial or total removal of the clitoris and labia minora with or without excision of the labia majora
3. Narrowing the vaginal orifice with creation of a covering seal by cutting and appositioning the labia minor and/or labia majora, with or without excision of the clitoris.
4. Unclassified – can include pricking or incising of the clitoris or labia or introduction of corrosive substances or herbs into the vagina.

The reasons for FGM vary according to the community it is being practised in, but the World Health Organization uses the following list to consider the most prevalent:

1. Where FGM is a social convention (social norm), the social pressure to conform to what others do and have been doing, as well as the need to be accepted socially and the fear of being rejected by the community, are strong motivations to perpetuate the practice. In some communities, FGM is almost universally performed and unquestioned.

2. FGM is often considered a necessary part of raising
   a girl, and a way to prepare her for adulthood and
   marriage.
3. FGM is often motivated by beliefs about what is
   considered acceptable sexual behaviour. It aims
   to ensure premarital virginity and marital fidelity.
   FGM is in many communities believed to reduce
   a woman's libido and therefore believed to help
   her resist extramarital sexual acts. When a vaginal
   opening is covered or narrowed (type 3), the fear
   of the pain of opening it, and the fear that this
   will be found out, is expected to further discourage
   extramarital sexual intercourse among women with
   this type of FGM.
4. Where it is believed that being cut increases
   marriageability, FGM is more likely to be carried
   out.
5. FGM is associated with cultural ideals of femininity
   and modesty, which include the notion that girls are
   clean and beautiful after removal of body parts that
   are considered unclean, unfeminine or male.[22]

While no religious texts specifically endorse FGM, practitioners will often justify it as being supported by religion.
Religious leaders take widely divergent positions, from
actively promoting it, to regarding it as irrelevant, both
culturally and spiritually, to campaigning for its elimination.
But local authority figures and community leaders, including
those actively involved, such as circumcisers or medical
personnel, may work hard to retain the practice.

A study in Sudan has shown that girls who have undergone

FGM are at risk of infertility in subsequent years because of recurring infections.[23] Lars Almroth, a paediatrician from the Karolina Institute in Stockholm, led the study: 'Children are bedridden for at least a week following mutilation and suffer immediate complications and infections of the reproductive system, and repeated urinary tract infections that often lead to kidney failure. But very, very few make it to hospital. As a result, the untreated infections of childhood ascend to the uterus and fallopian tubes, causing scarring, inflammation and infertility. A pre-pubescent girl's vaginal [tract] is a low protective oestrogenic environment, and the lack of vaginal acidity in these young girls allows the bacteria to thrive . . . Changes in the microfauna that result means the vaginal environment may become unfavourable to sperm, and also less able to guard against constant infection leading to further inflammation – all of which reduces fertility.'[24]

In Sudan a woman's value is heavily dependent on her ability to be a mother; an infertile woman can find herself rejected by her husband and kin as well as by wider society. The study, which had 279 subjects, provided medical evidence of a correlation between primary infertility and FGM and it was hoped that awareness of how the practice affected the possibility of motherhood might help in the campaign to abolish the practice.[25]

Another recent study in Kenya considers the relationship between FGM and obstetric fistula.[26] If childbirth is prolonged, a child may become stuck in the birthing canal and a hole or fistula may develop between the vagina and the bladder and/or rectum. This can cause urinary and faecal incontinence. Lilian Mwanri and Glory Gatwiri, from Flinders University, Australia, highlight the cases of three women.

Twenty-two-year-old Sasha, from Samburu in northern
Kenya, was married at the age of nine, just after her FGM
ceremony. 'You know, in Samburu, it is expected that you
will do this thing. They took me early in the morning and
poured really cold water on me. It was so painful but I was
not allowed to scream . . .'[27] Sasha fell pregnant when she
was eleven. Her labour lasted for six terrible days and at the
end she gave birth to a dead, macerated baby. Afterwards
she collapsed. When she came round she smelled her own
bodily waste and realized she was doubly incontinent.
'When I developed this problem [fistula] and came to
this hospital, one of the nurses said that this thing [FGM]
and the way it was done had contributed to me having
this urine problem.'[28] Sasha's husband left her and took
another wife. She suffers not only from the after-effects of
the birth but is also vulnerable to the ridicule and disdain
of her neighbours, both because of her embarrassing
condition, and because she is without a husband or child.
'Especially when the urine passes, it burns you so much you
turn completely red . . . When you say or do something,
they tell you to go away with your urine or your faeces.
My husband would tell me that I would for ever leak urine,
that it would never go away. It would make me feel like I
wanted to die.'[29]

One of the most interesting features of Sasha's and
the other women's accounts is that, until the medical staff
told them that their problems were in part attributable to
FGM, they did not make the connection. Women who
are complicit in the practice may not be fully aware of the
medical consequences of the procedure that was performed
on them when they were very young, and which they may

in turn have done to their daughters. Mwanri and Gatwiri's study demonstrates that, because of 'power imbalances and marginalization of women, FGM is practised without considering the harmful impacts it can cause on women and those surrounding them.'[30] Because the process may be romanticized within the culture, it is essential that women are made more aware of the possible consequences. As in Sudan, Kenyan society also places a very high value on a woman's ability to bear children. Perhaps the risk to fertility caused directly or indirectly by FGM will in time help to develop new understanding within traditional communities and eradicate the practice altogether.

Those Who Were Denied by the State

Chinese cultural practice and the one-child policy, which was enforced from 1979 and is only now, in the past decade, being phased out, have led to a disparity between male and female populations which means that at the time of writing there are some 30 million Chinese men who remain unmarried and childless. For those in poor, rural communities their state can also add to economic hardship.

The country's rapid economic growth is well documented, as is the cost to some in society who are no longer included in village life. During the collectivization period that began in the 1950s, economic resources and working roles were controlled and distributed by the collective. Jobs would be assigned to those most suited to them, so an elderly or infirm person would still work but at a task that was lighter or better suited to his or her abilities. The elderly who were childless, and therefore had no family to provide another source of income, would get priority for such jobs, with loans of grain and other forms of support in times of need. But the late 1970s brought marketization. While this meant greater wealth for many villages and towns, these new-found riches did not benefit everyone in society equally. Local government focused far more of the available funds on communities or families who could influence their re-election.

Traditionally in Chinese society a son is considered preferable to a daughter, so, with the restriction on having only one child, female children were frequently aborted, adopted or even killed in the hope that the next child might be a boy. Female infanticide was historically part of Chinese culture but its prevalence in the late twentieth century, at odds with the Communist Party's focus on gender equality, is a result of the one-child policy.[31]

Compliance was promoted through a system of punishment and reward. The preference for a sole child to be male was especially marked in farming communities, where male offspring were seen as better suited to the heavy agricultural labour that provided the family income, but it also reflected the fact that a daughter would usually go to her in-laws, while a son would remain part of his birth family, able to contribute to his parents' well-being in their old age. By 1982, the Chinese press was publishing accounts of parents killing girl infants and of women being abused because they had borne daughters. In 1987 a fine of 2,000 yuan was imposed on any illegal birth in southern Guangdong but would be diminished to 300 yuan if the infant died within three months. Julie Jimmerson, from the UCLA School of Law, observes that 'parents could conceivably kill an illegal infant daughter to try again later for a son, and pay only a fraction of the fine'.[32] She quotes a township director as saying, 'No one wants to pay a fine for a girl.'

Abortions based on sex were illegal but well attested throughout the country, since ultrasound scans made fore-knowledge of gender possible. Infant girls would be aban-doned in streets and alleyways, parks and at the doors of local institutions; parents kept their birth a secret, hop-ing for a male child to carry the family line. But while the 'dying rooms' of Chinese orphanages – the places of neglect and abandonment where female babies and toddlers were consigned to slow deaths – became notorious through inter-national media and journalism, another minority group was also being created in their wake.

By the year 2000, the gender discrepancy, the legacy of murder and abandonment, was having significant demo-graphic impact. In some provinces, such as Anhui, Jiangxi and Shaanxi, more than 130 male children were being born for every 100 female children. The men who remain unmarried and childless tend to be the poorest in society or those who suffer from physical or mental disabilities. Their vulnerability is then compounded by having no offspring to care for them or to share any improved prosperity. These are the surplus men, isolated in a society where welfare provision ranges from sporadic and disorganized to non-existent, and where families are expected to take care of their own.

Academic papers can be a conduit for stories, but often the personal details are hidden behind impersonal language, figures and tables. Weiguo Zhang's 2007 study of China's surplus men is an exception because it is neither dispassionate nor arid.[33] In the village he discusses, the only people considered to be so poor that they were in need of help were all elderly childless men. Village elders were not unaware of the isolation and loneliness that the men suffered; one Communist Party official told the visiting academics, 'Nobody would even know if they had died at home!'

Malong was a short man, something that both he and many villagers believed had made it difficult for him to find a wife. All four of his siblings, two younger, two older, were dead. His house had no heating system at all. It was hidden by overgrown vegetation that filled his small yard, connected to the village by a slender path, hidden from view, ignored. He had no money to improve his home because his only source of income was to work the land that was contracted to him and he was too frail to do so. Instead, a niece from an adjacent village worked the land for him. While she kept all of the produce and the resulting income for her own family, she did cook food for him every few days and bring it to him. He wasn't able to prepare his own food but sometimes he would exchange some of his small store of corn or wheat for the steamed bread that was sold by peddlers going door to door.

It was an imperfect system; he once had no food for seven days, had nothing but water with vinegar, because his niece was ill. Malong was reliant on neighbours for water and, apart from a local Christian representative who occasionally visited with food, his only other interaction was with a group of school children who liked to come to his house. The young people listened to his stories of Communism, and, according to the village officials, brought food and sometimes wine or cigarettes from their parents' houses without their permission. The officials didn't like Malong's recollections of the past, saying he was not teaching 'good stuff' to his visitors. So the visits were stopped and Malong returned to his rarely interrupted isolation, within the walls of his hidden house. He told the researchers: 'Nobody cares about you. People see you as dirty, and being able to do nothing. In the past old people who reached sixty would be left alone in a well. Those children who were filial might leave some food for you. Gradually the old would die. That occurred hundreds of years ago. Nobody bothers about you now. You can live as long as 100 years! Nobody cares.'

Laofang lived in the same village. His siblings, two elder brothers and sisters and a younger sister, were all dead. There was extended family – nephews and nieces, great nephews and nieces – but not in the immediate vicinity. They visited him when they could, bringing food and often spending the Spring Festival and Dragon Festival with him. Laofang's health was good too, except in winter, when chronic bronchitis flared up. He had a good appetite, could move around the village, was even able to do some of the tasks on his contracted land, such as watering the crops and other lighter duties. But one of his nephews had to do the more strenuous work for him, such as sowing, ploughing fields, harvesting the crop, in return taking more than half of what was grown as payment. The remainder was insufficient for even a basic standard of living, but Laofang also kept three sheep at a time and could feed them by gathering weeds and grass from the fields on a daily basis; in the autumn the sale of the sheep supplemented his income.

Laofang recounted his life simply, explaining that he awoke at six or seven in the morning, made his food, collected the food for the sheep, perhaps walked in the village. He went to sleep at eight or nine in the evening, fully dressed, more napping than sleeping, just in case anyone tried to steal his sheep. His house was simple, had remained unchanged since the 1960s and the collectivization period, although other places in the village had been modernized, renovated. There was a coal stove to heat the bedroom in wintertime and an electric light bulb, which the visiting academic noted was seldom on, except for a few hours in the late evening, so the house was almost always shadowy or dark. This puzzled the academic, because Laofang did not pay for his electricity.

To me it was less strange; it made me think of my mother. Since Dad's death, she's alone in our council house in Scotland and is careful with switching on the ceiling lights, simply because when one bulb runs out, she has to worry about finding someone to change it, at least between our frequent visits.

The universality of dependence that links Laofang with my mother connects us all. There is the question of what obligation the state has, and what we owe to each other. Any state support we have is a cobweb-like thing, easily destroyed, but strong in what it is able to do. And in cultures where support does not exist, or is unregulated or patchy, there is nothing but the obligation of children to ease the later years. Without that, there is only the kindness of strangers.

But while financial security in old age, whether for the childless or not, is an issue to some degree in all societies, the emotional problems vary in different countries and cultures. Studies report that in China older adults show significantly higher levels of loneliness, depression and lower life satisfaction than in the West, even when economic factors are strictly controlled.[34]

In 2013 the Communist Party finally announced a lessening of the one-child policy. Two years later, the Chinese leaders went further, spurred on by international comment, perhaps, and began to try to make amends for the policy that had changed the demographic of the country. In June 2015 the China Daily News Service reported on the creation of the No. 5 Welfare Nursing Home in Beijing. A high-end nursing home that welcomed the aged elite of the city, new and future residents would be only those who had had a single child in accordance with the one-child policy but then suffered the death of that only offspring. Official statistics reported by the press showed that in 2013 alone there were 8,781 senior residents of Beijing in that position. This newest initiative aimed to provide not only physical comfort and security but also emotional support for those who find themselves childless in their later years.

Yet the cultural stigma of childlessness, especially in rural communities, is not waning. Ancestor worship, having been abandoned during the Communist period, is resurging again. Its long tradition stretches back to the oracle bones discovered at Anyang, dating from 1600 BC, which allowed ancestors to guide and warn future generations, and the *Analects of Confucius* from the fourth century BC. Accounts from the twenty-first century attest to renewed ancestor veneration in provinces across China.[35] To have children is to increase the clan; to fail to do so is to break a chain of worship that can go back for a thousand years.[36] And even where the practice is no longer followed, its legacy remains in stigmatization and neglectful policy. Thus, despite the welcome improvement of a comfortable place for grieving parents to pass their last years, the question that remains for the state is how to make a path of possibility for the forgotten Chinese, those who never had any children at all.

A Short Note on the Naming of Names

Stories are precious things. Some long to be heard and wish to be shouted, proclaimed, owned by their teller. Others told in distorted voices set in unfamiliar places, peopled by imaginary names.

Often, with grant-enabled academic research, strict anonymity can be a condition of publication. In the course of writing this book I spoke to at least one academic who felt frustrated by this rule, who said, over and over, I wish I could tell you where my informants are so that you might go, hear more, share their world with another audience. It is what they wanted themselves.

The choice of identity in this book always lies with the teller of the tale. Sur's family, in their small village in India, afraid of gossip and possible censure, wished to be unidentifiable from even the smallest detail. In contrast, the women of Gambaga, in Ghana, gave their stories to the film-maker Yaba Badoe because they wished to be heard, discussed for who they are and were. When I retold them, I was asked to honour this wish and was glad to do so.

In a pause, think of Mary Osuma, condemned to the witches' camp in Gambaga – imagine her life, cast out from her home and her family, named as an evil, ill-wishing, supernatural creature. In Mary's last years, her brothers did come for her, took her home; for Mary there was some respite in later life. Then think too of the Bolivian phone lines, arterial voices murmuring across continents, connecting silenced women with kindness and the wish to help. Of the girl called Sur, who is not Sur, but someone just like her. Of the named men and women who all wanted to own their experiences, and of those others who wanted to tell but to do so in disguised voices, under assumed names.

Listen. Remember. In doing so we are beginning to defy.

A Short Note on Things That Matter

When I was small, I used to call my mother's female friends my aunts. They were kindly women who sent me little gifts and added drawings of cats for me at the bottom of their letters to my mother.

When one of my closest friends invited me to be god-mother to his daughter, I was pleased, not only because I felt honoured, but because it meant I had a role in Hannah's life. I had been given a title. I was to be her godmother – not just her dad's friend, but someone connected *to* her.

I am not a mother. I will never be a grandmother. I am not a sister. I am a wife and a daughter and a niece. I am a godmother to Hannah. It is a defining thing. My mother's friends were not defined in any way by their relationship with me. To be a godmother matters.

The christening was an intimate one in an Anglican church in Rotterdam, where Hannah's parents, Michael and Lena, live. But it was the following day, sitting in a sandpit with Hannah, building a castle of sorts, which we decorated with feather and stones, that I really thought about being part of her life.

In medieval Europe spiritual kinship could be used to political and economic advantage. By the ninth century, the titles endowed at a christening related the godparent not just to the christened infant but to the parents themselves, as a co-parent. Sexual taboos and marriage bans surrounded these fictive familial relations, and a child would have spiritual siblings (if the God/co parent had children) as well as spiritual in-laws. Historically the godparent's function was both spiritual and pragmatic. Godparenting was seen as equal to parenting, and often childless women were asked to perform the role. Between 1553 and 1555, childless Anna Bauer was godmother to 57 children.[1] In seventeenth-century France childless godparents would often adopt their godchildren officially, taking them to live in their homes and bring them up as their own children, especially when their parents could not afford to support a large family.[2]

Anthropologists use the term 'fictive kin' to describe kinship that does not have blood or marriage links; it is in opposition to true kinship. Fictive kin, like a childless woman, is defined by what it does not have. Personally, the phrase irks me – the implication that truth should somehow depend on sanguineous ties, or that the ceremony of marriage can create 'real' kinship while the ceremony of christening cannot.

Nowadays the role of godparent is still ostensibly to watch over a Christian upbringing, but in practice it has many other facets. Hannah's mother, Lena, spoke to me of her own godparents, of how important they were to her; she described them as a continuity in her life and said she wished the same for her daughter. For her, it was not principally the traditional Christian side of the role but rather the friendship and constancy it could bring. I do not have godparents. My parents believed that anything that took place in a church should only take place once I was old enough to decide for myself if I had faith or not. For Lena, the role was something else, a kind of official friendship. For my friend Michael, beyond the traditional religious role, there was also a sense of welcoming someone new into the family of his youngest daughter. We have been friends for more than thirty years, never lost touch, never ceased to be involved in each other's lives, even when we were geographically very distant. Perhaps the formalizing of my relationship to Hannah should not matter, but it does. I feel less childless because of it.

4

Those Who Adapt

People find myriad ways of adapting to life in cultures where the bias against the childless is marked. Some adaptations are overt and defiant, some stealthy or designed to placate the anger of society, others are about recovering worth and respect. Some may be personal, not public – secrets kept to preserve hope or possibility – or they may be shared openly and recognized by the society. There are unusual collaborations, developed to mutual benefit, and there are webs of deception involving complicit and sympathetic family members. Many marginalized infertile men and women no longer wish to be seen as victims of their circumstances. Instead they present themselves as bravely defying stereotypes by means of quiet resistance, socio-economic ingenuity, innovative alliances and redefined cultural identities.

Resistance in Any Circumstances

Chandni, a student of English, from Dhaka, in Bangladesh, was expecting her first child. Over a three-year period, she had undergone a series of alternative and traditional medical treatments to help her to conceive, but each of them had been kept secret from her husband. Chandni's marriage was not an unhappy one; on the contrary, these clandestine appointments, made possible with the collusion of her mother and sister, were the result of love. Chandni was afraid her husband's parents would make him take a second wife if she was unable to conceive after the first years of their marriage. But within Bangladeshi culture, it is only acceptable to take another bride when all attempts at fertility treatment have failed. Had she not fallen pregnant, Chandni would have begun fertility treatment to buy more time from her husband and his family.

Bangladesh is a patriarchal society and a childless woman, especially one born in a rural area, may be disdained and stigmatized for her inability to perform her prime function, which is to be a bearer of sons. The issue of infertility is often overlooked because the country is overpopulated, and population control has been a government priority since 1976.[1] Infertility is also not recognized as a health issue, and therefore medical treatment and support is difficult to access. Patriarchal social structures result in marked gender inequality and a woman's only value may be seen as her ability to produce healthy male children. For a woman who fails to have a child, the issues are 'social, familial, emotional, economic and medical' and she will be labelled as 'deviant'.[2] Immediately after her wedding, a woman is expected to move into her husband's parental home, and within the year may find that her new husband and his family conspire in physical and mental abuse if she does not become pregnant.

With little to no obvious control over their circumstances, such women may be stereotyped as passive, victims of their culture and circumstances. Yet even in this environment, where any attempt at resistance would be fraught with difficulty and risk, Bangladeshi women try to manage their situation, to adapt, resist and even confront the stigmatization.[3]

Kabery was married at the age of twenty-five. She used to be quiet and withdrawn when asked about her lack of children. Her inability to conceive made her embarrassed and reluctant to engage: 'There was a time when I could not say anything when somebody asked me about children, I just remained silent and sad and came home and cried.'[4] Now she feels that she is 'strong enough to face this question and find a way that people will not ask me about it any more'. Kabery has gained confidence in her own worth. 'Now if people ask, "Why don't you have a child?" I sharply answer them. I just say to them, "What can I do about it, should I make a baby with clay and show you?"'[5]

Kabery and Chandni are both urbanites; for rural women in Bangladesh, circumstances can be even more difficult to navigate. They often have little or no independent finances, which are controlled by men, and their sphere of influence is small. However, they are generally in charge of preparing food for the household. Food becomes their currency and, by keeping a little aside each day, they are able to sell it to beggars and itinerants and thus accumulate a little cash to pay for herbal or conventional medicine. A woman who was married at sixteen but was still childless after five years saved enough money to buy a goat by selling scraps of food. She now keeps the goat at her mother's home and saves the profits from the sale of its milk so that she can eventually afford fertility treatment.[6]

Collaboration and Association

Internationally, an established way of reacting to stigma-tization is to form a public group or association of people who share your experience. In recent years, in developed countries these have often become virtual societies that aim to bring childless men and women together in the hope that they may find strength in solidarity, support to face the issues caused by their shared situation. But elsewhere in the world these groups are often physical points of reference for women from diverse local communities, safe spaces where they can speak of their personal experience and be listened to.

The groups may come together by accident or design. One year after a joint research project by Harvard University and the Bulgarian Academy of Sciences on 'women's resistive voices' in the context of childlessness in Bulgaria, the women who had been interviewed formed an advocacy organization.[7] This group began by presenting infertility as a medical condition and fighting for access to effective and affordable treatment. Through advocacy, it hoped to regulate fertility clinics as well as develop a way of evaluating their success, with better subsidies from the government to support fertility treatment. The idea of combatting stigma was not a primary goal, but instead the group's members supported each other in achieving better ways of improving the treatment available to them.[8]

In the Yakurr community in southern Nigeria, societies for women are a fundamental part of life, with many cultural groups and church-based associations. Until a decade ago, one such society, the Kekonakona, offered a place for infertile women to gather and share their difficulties and experience.

Its primary focus, like the Bulgarian group, was to help its members conceive, but beyond that it acted as an informal support for the childless and enabled them to take part more fully in community life. Now the number of members has dwindled significantly, a phenomenon that reflects the growing popularity of evangelical Christianity in the region. The two facts are not coincidental. Younger women explain that they have no interest in joining such a group because it is at odds with their faith, while one woman adds, 'I would never join the Kekonakona because its members have to appear bare-breasted in certain public rituals,' which was at odds with her modern sensibilities and sense of Christian decorum.[9]

But fertility is no less an issue, so, in keeping with their new beliefs, women are increasingly turning to the 'power of prayer' rather than to each other. Frustrated by the cost of medical infertility treatments, they regard their lack of children as a problem that can only be solved with God's intervention.

Unlike the majority of such groups in Africa, the main focus of Zimbabwe's Chipo Chedu Society is not to campaign for access to infertility treatment, or to support women during it, but instead to tackle the issues surrounding the stigmatizing of childlessness in the culture. It was founded by Betty Chishava in 1996 as a result of her own experience of the ostracism and humiliation suffered by women who cannot conceive.[10] In Zimbabwe an infertile woman suffers severe societal rejection and is regarded as inadequate. Male infertility, on the other hand, is rarely discussed. On the rare occasions when it is acknowledged within the family, it may be concealed from others by secretly bringing in a relative of the husband, often his brother, to impregnate his wife. Chishava herself almost fell victim to this practice when her parents, despairing of her lack of offspring, tried to arrange for her husband's brother to have sex with her. Chishava refused, saying that it was against her Christian beliefs. Many Zimbabwean women turn to sleeping with multiple partners, despite the high risk of HIV, in the hope that one such encounter will leave them carrying a child. Some women turn to faith healers. Chishava chose to question these ways of dealing with the problem, because she felt that the real issue was a cultural one. She set out to challenge the prejudice and discrimination within her society that made women feel they had to resort to any means available in order to have a child. She formed a group with three other women in the same position and together they conducted a survey to ascertain the scale and scope of Zimbabwean female infertility, reaching the conclusion that around 5 per cent of women had failed to fall pregnant while in a heterosexual relationship. Further research conducted in four of the country's ten provinces then identified possible coping mechanisms for women that they might support. The reception was overwhelming, with the women surveyed identifying their need for social and economic empowerment within their respective communities.[11]

The name 'Chipo Chedu' means 'our own gift', reflecting an acceptance of infertility. Chishava organizes courses for women to learn skills that will enable them to support themselves if their husbands leave them as a result of their inability to have children. In a bid for funding in 2017, she explained that childless women 'have never organized, partly because most have internalized a debilitating shame that leads them to withdraw from the public eye'.[12] Today the society employs forty-two women in small towns around Zimbabwe. When women have lost any support from their families and communities, Chishava listens. 'I talk to women about the nature of their relationships, whether their partner beats them, why they believe they haven't conceived, their feelings on adoption, if they've ever visited a specialist, or attended counselling or skills training workshops . . . We have staged dramas with follow-up discussion sessions all around the country. In rural areas I have tried to educate communities to assist childless couples by integrating them in all activities rather than neglecting them.'[13]

In Britain the charity Fertility Network UK offers support and guidance to both genders. There are opportunities to form groups and forums and meet other people in similar situations. There are also suggestions for coping strategies, ways of adapting your life to help deal with some of the emotional and practical difficulties, formulated into a toolkit which suggests going through a grieving process, something that is often mentioned by experts on childlessness as being part of recovery – the idea that you have to acknowledge a loss before moving on with your new life. But there are also recommendations that echo the experience of Kabery in Bangladesh, such as learning to say, 'No, I don't have children', and then regaining control of the conversation that follows.[14]

One international online community that brings together women who are involuntarily childless so that they can support and comfort each other is the Dovecote. Their Facebook forum is a virtual safe space where women confide in strangers who share their circumstances about the difficulties they face. Often these are the kind of experiences that are difficult to voice elsewhere: the wish to avoid children because of the pain they can bring, or family disagreements that cannot be discussed in a small local community without the confider feeling disloyal. The group was created by Kelly Da Silva as a result of her own experience of infertility, with the aim of helping individuals as well as changing society's perceptions. I drop in on the Facebook page from time to time. I read the stories of the women and I too find comfort in the similarity of experience, the act of sharing. Paradoxically, this forum for those who are involuntarily childless is a place where wisdom and experience are passed down from one generation to another. The messages of how we have coped or what we have suffered and survived may comfort those who read them, but there is also pride in giving that comfort, a sense of value regained.

Despite the very disparate nature of these groups, there is a commonality that offers hope. The similarity of coping mechanisms, across communities and cultures, hints at a future of shared understanding extending beyond each personal experience. With ever increasing access to the internet across the globe, and fewer problems caused by physical distance, the lack of a common spoken language, rather than cultural differences, may be the biggest barrier to creating a group that embraces our diverse circumstances but offers support across the divide.

Cultural Adaptations

Keqi became a *burrnesha*, or 'sworn virgin', when she was just twenty. She is one of a small group of childless women in northern Albania who continue to live their lives in a way dictated by centuries-old law.

In a decision made somewhere between choice and necessity, the *burrnesha* have taken a vow of chastity to live as men for the rest of their lives. The Albanian *Kanun* is a set of customary laws that has been passed down orally since the fifteenth century and was only committed to paper in the twentieth. The laws govern all aspects of life, from economy to marriage to land governance. There are also rules governing how crime is to be addressed, and adherence to these, in parts of rural Albania, led to blood feuds that perpetuated themselves over generations, resulting in revenge killings and isolation for those who feared becoming victims. One way of ending a long-running feud was by an arranged marriage; the only way the bride could escape this marriage and not reignite the dispute was to swear to live as a *burrnesha*. But escaping an unwanted union was not the only reason that women chose to become 'sworn virgins'. The prevalence of honour killings in northern Albanian society meant that families could be left without any male members. In this situation an elder daughter might choose to become a *burrnesha* to act as the man of her household. She would be treated as a man within the community, enjoy the freedom afforded to men, but also represent her family in any continuation of the feud. The custom is vanishing, and few, if any, women become *burrnesha* today, but a handful or so still live in the remote mountains of Albania, largely wary of outsiders and attention.[15]

Keqi's father had been murdered in a blood feud, and the other men in the family, her four brothers, had openly opposed Enver Hoxha's Communist regime and were in prison or dead. Taking a vow of celibacy and committing to live as a man enabled Keqi to support her mother, her four sisters-in-law and their five children.[16] Keqi worked in construction and even prayed at the mosque with local men: 'I was totally free as a man, because no one knew I was a woman. I could go wherever I wanted to and no one would dare swear at me because I could beat them up. I was only with men. I don't know how to do women's talk. I am never scared.'[17]

As a man, Keqi had to avenge her father's death, and when her father's killer was released from prison at the age of eighty, she ordered her nephew to kill him. But his death led to more retaliation, with his family killing Keqi's nephew in revenge. 'I always dreamed of avenging my father's death. My brothers tried to, but did not succeed. Of course, I have regrets my nephew was killed. But if you kill me, I have to kill you.'[18] Today Keqi lives in Tirania. The true patriarch of her extended family, her nieces will never marry without her permission. She says that she does not regret that she is childless because she is surrounded by her nephews and nieces, and sees a lack of sexual relations as the sacrifice she had no choice but to make.[19]

The position of women in Albanian society is improving; the surviving *burrnesha* are in their seventies and eighties. Keqi reminisces that in her younger days a woman and an animal had the same worth, but says that 'Now Albanian women have equal rights with men and are even more powerful, and I think today it would be fun to be a woman.'[20]

In order to gain control of their lives and protect those around them, to be freed from the restrictions of their patriarchal culture, Keqi, like other women in her community, changed their social gender to the dominant one. Professor Linda Gusia from the University of Pristina in Kosovo comments that 'Stripping off their sexuality by pledging to remain virgins was a way for these women in a male-dominated, segregated society to engage in public life. It was about surviving in a world where men rule.'[21]

Those Who Adapt: Dying to be Accepted

Most of the accommodations discussed so far have been made possible through networks, whether it is the mother who hides the goat in Bangladesh, or a normally conservative society colluding in and accepting a gender change to meet a family's needs or position. These strategies look to future life and possibility, are ways of managing existing societies or trying to change them. Other darker options exist, where a childlessness woman may believe that the worthlessness of her life can be overcome only by her sacrifice.

Wafa Idris was in her late twenties. Her husband had divorced her after nine years of marriage because, following a stillbirth, she was informed that she would never carry a baby to term. She had been returned to her parents, an economic burden, with no status and no possibility of gaining any within the male-dominated society of Palestine. On 27 January 2002, dressed in her paramedic uniform, she drove a Red Crescent ambulance through the main checkpoint between the West Bank and Jerusalem. The vehicle carried a backpack filled with a ten-kilo bomb. It may be that Idris originally intended to pass the bag to another terrorist, but plans somehow changed, so that it was she who carried it to Jaffa Street, in central Jerusalem, and detonated it outside a shoe shop. It killed Idris herself and an Israeli man named Pinhas Tokatli, who was shown by worldwide media burning in flames, and injured over a hundred people.

Idris was the first female suicide bomber in Israel and she very quickly became a martyr; media coverage far surpassed that of any of the male suicide bombers who had gone before her. No longer regarded as an unmarriageable childless woman, in death she was hailed as a heroine. The Iraqi president, Saddam Hussein, ordered a memorial in Baghdad to honour her. In Egypt the television producer Dr Amira Abu-Fatuh paid tribute to Idris with a television programme, and the weekly publication *Saut-Al-Umma* declared: 'Wafa Idris elevated the value of the Arab woman and, in one moment, and with enviable courage, put an end to the unending debate about equality between men and women.'[22]

Her posthumous reputation within much of the Arab-speaking world was in marked contrast to the position she held in her society when alive. Palestinian journalist Budour Hassan describes the gender discrimination within Palestinian 'patriarchal society', where 'divorced women are often dehumanized and treated like scourges and onerous burdens'.[23] Between 1991 and 2013, 162 Palestinian women behind the Green Line were murdered by their husbands or other family members, despite Israel's ratification of the Convention on the Elimination of All Forms of Discrimination against Women. The situation continues to get worse.

In the first nine months of 2016, thirteen women were killed either by family members or by contracted killers.[24] In 2017, in protest at the scale of the problem, 12,000 people signed a petition for Mahmoud Abbas, president of the Palestinian Authority, organized by Palestinian women's groups. It called for a change in the Jordanian penal code, which operates in Palestine and, the groups claim, allows the perpetrators of so called 'honour' killings to receive reduced sentences.[25]

Idris's political conviction was promoted as the motivation for her act, but it may be only part of her narrative. Dr Mira Tzoreff, from Tel Aviv University, argues that 'She was non-formative in Palestinian society and her chances of building a new life for herself were close to zero. Wafa Idris's only way of redeeming herself was by choosing to become a Shahida for the sake of her nation.'[26]

A few journalists in the Arab press also rejected the notion of solely political motivation. The *Asharq al-Awsat* newspaper presented Idris's biography and speculated that her inability to have a child combined with her divorce may have led to her terrorist act. In doing so, they were questioning not only her motivation but the very nature of the act: to depoliticize the motive is to say that the women are not terrorists at all.

Idris's situation and that of the other female bomber, Dareen Abu Aysheh, who followed immediately in her wake, reflected the call of the First Intifada, from 1987 to 1993, which had urged women to give birth to soldiers. Article 17 of the Hamas Charter of 1988 stated: 'The Muslim woman has a role in the struggle for liberation that does not fall from that of the man in that she is the one who produced the men.'[27] Now Idris had opened up another possibility for those who were not, or could not become, mothers – that of joining the cause and acting as a suicide bomber.

The second female Palestinian suicide bomber, a childless twenty-one-year-old student, went beyond the idea of self-sacrifice and sought to inspire other attacks, couching her declaration in a birth metaphor: 'Let Sharon the coward know that every Palestinian woman will give birth to an army of martyrs, and her role will not only be confined to weeping over a son, brother or husband; instead, she will become a martyr herself.'[28] Yet in marked contrast, the man who arranged her martyrdom, Nasser Shawish of Fatah, was initially opposed to her decision, saying in interviews with Yoram Schweitzer, head of Israel's Institute for National Security Studies, that 'She was a pretty and successful girl, studying at the university, a future mother, who should marry and bear many children.'[29]

Then, for the first time, in 2004, a female bomber who was also a mother, Rim Riashi, blew herself up at the Erez checkpoint, taking the lives of four Israeli soldiers. She left two young children and a husband. Yet her motive was far from purely political; it transpired her illicit relationship with a lover had become known and gossiped about locally, staining her family honour. Her suicide redeemed not only herself but her family name.[30]

After Idris's death, the London Arab newspaper *Al Quds Al-Arabi* quoted the Fatah Revolutionary Council as saying, 'The martyr's death of Wafa restored honour to the national role of Palestinian women'.[31] With Riashi's death, however, the celebration was more hesitant; dialogue and debate followed, with Fatah even questioning the use of women in the role: 'A twenty-two-year-old girl, mother of two children, one of them a baby and the other a little girl, carried out an act of self-sacrifice. Who issued a Muslim religious ruling depriving the baby of its mother? On the basis of which passages in the Qur'an and the Hadith does a young mother abandon her true jihad role, which is raising two children, one of whom needs milk?'[32] This was in direct contrast with the previous media storm, which had largely focused on how the acts of female suicide bombers brought them not only redemption and honour, but also equality with men. The childless bombers had proved their worth to a society that did not value them in life, but even death and killing could not restore them to their 'true jihad role': that of a mother.

During the civil war in Sri Lanka, which ended in 2009, the Liberation Tigers of Tamil Elam (LTTE) had both male and female combat units, including those for suicide bombers. The bombers were known as Black Tigers, with the women often being dubbed Black Tigresses in the press. The first spate of bombers were childless and generally un-married, leading to the claim that their sacrifice was like an extension of the notion of motherhood in Hindu Tamil culture, whereby a Tamil mother would sacrifice herself for her natural sons. The co-ordinator of the organization Women for Peace, Silva Mangalika, admitted: 'Acting as a human bomb is an understood and accepted offering for a woman who will never be a mother.'[33]

The first LTTE female suicide bomber was a Tamil teenager, Dhanu, who succeeded in killing the Indian prime minister, Rajiv Gandhi, in May 1991. She was childless and a minor. some media sources claimed at the time that she had agreed to the act in revenge for an alleged rape by the

Indian Peace Keeping Force, although it is unclear if this was factual or LTTE propaganda.

In 2008 *Marie Claire* magazine gained an exclusive interview with a Black Tiger who had been arrested after a failed suicide attempt. If successful, it would have resulted in the killing of the then Sri Lankan prime minister, Ratnasiri Wickremanayake.[34] Menake was twenty-seven and her terrorist identity was discovered because of her cyanide necklace, a capsule that all LTTE members wear round their necks to take in the event of capture. In common with many bombers, Menake had been a rape victim. When she was seven, her alcoholic father had raped her repeatedly for four days. The forced loss of virginity makes such women unmarriageable; the act of killing gives them both respect and the possibility of purification by fire, in keeping with Hindu ritual.

Her grandfather rescued her from her abusive father and, when he died, her aunt and uncle took her in. By 2000, the LTTE needed more recruits and ordered Tamils to donate one male or female family member to its ranks. Seeing her as nothing but a burden, Menake's relatives offered her up. Menake recounts that she volunteered to be a Black Tiger because she was depressed and saw no future for herself. She was also in pain from spinal nerve damage and had been told she might be paralyzed when she was older. 'I thought, why continue to live? A lot of girls were volunteering to be suicide bombers, so I thought I would too.'

In Tamil the word for suicide mission is *thatkodai*, 'gift of self'; for Menake, it meant her life had meaning.[35] She was told she would be given great honour after her death. However, she was not without sadness: 'If I felt sad, it was because I would never have the opportunity to have a family and children, to hold my own baby in my arms. That was my biggest sorrow.'

The *Marie Claire* journalist asked an LTTE spokesman how he justified sending young women to kill in this way, and he replied that he saw them not as killers but as givers. For him too, perhaps, it was another way of giving for those who could not give birth.

Those Who Adapt:
Woman to Woman Marriage

In many parts of the African continent, motherhood is often the sole way in which a woman can develop her status within a social group or community. In some instances, the shame of childlessness is so extreme as to result in social exclusion and isolation, in much the way that it does in the Indian cases already discussed. Research from Mozambique, Nigeria and Ghana shows childless women being forbidden from attending festivals, celebrations and community gatherings, even shunned because of the bad luck associated with their state. A Ghanaian study, focused on a group of Muslim women, showed that the depression rate was extremely high, perhaps reflecting the importance of childbearing within the faith, and the fact that it could lead to family disharmony, and to an unwanted second wife being introduced.[36] This differed from my own, admittedly unscientific, conversations in Qatar, where bigamy, and the children it might bring to the household, was seen by some as a blessing. But then I remembered the wary sidestepping of Noor, her surprised

disappointment at her husband's second marriage; I thought
how it would be impossible not to be depressed, when the
only thing that might break the cycle was beyond your
physical possibilities.

But in other parts of Africa, there are different ways of
getting a child – polygamy is only one possibility. Far more
unusual, far less discussed, is the idea of woman to woman
marriage. The practice does still exist today, although it is
less common, despite the fact that its legality continues to be
championed. A court case from 2011 allowed a woman married to another woman to inherit her late wife's property,
with the judge ruling that woman to woman marriage was a
recognized family institution in law.

In Kenya Lady Justice Ruth Sitati recently argued that
the 2010 constitution recognized traditional culture as 'the
foundation of the nation and as the cumulative civilization
of the Kenyan people and nation', meaning that woman
to woman marriage, a culturally accepted practice, was
recognized as legal and binding. She pointed out that 'Such
marriages reduced the scorn that was usually meted out by
society to women who has [sic] either given birth only to
daughters or not given birth to any children at all.' In her
summation Sitati concluded that the institution of woman to
woman marriage has an important place in Kenyan society,
'especially in view of the deeply embedded cultural beliefs
and practices about the importance of children in general
and sons in particular in society'.[37]

Years ago, I had been told of these weddings of women,
when I was working on Kikuyu, an agglutinative language
from Kenya, with an interesting phonological process called
Dahl's law. One of my Kikuyu informants had told me that

in his culture two women could marry, and often did so for
various reasons, the most common being childlessness. I lost
touch with him, but later recalled his half-joking remarks
about the Kikuyu being ahead of the west with their em-
bracing of woman to woman marriage. And it was not only
the Kikuyu who had the custom; since the beginning of the
twentieth century more than thirty different groups across
four sub-Saharan regions of Africa recorded incidences of
woman to woman marriage.[38]

Most of the Kuria group live around the Kenya-Tanzania
border, east of Lake Nyanza. There, a woman who marries
takes up her new life 'at the bottom of the hierarchy
and is certain to remain there if she fails to give birth to
children'.[39] Infertility is regarded as an ill omen; when a
woman dies childless, she is buried outwith the community
in an arid, lifeless place, a mirror of her own state, public
acknowledgement that she is *omogomba*, 'without offspring'.
The birth of a son is essential if a woman is to inherit on
the death of her husband. One way of overcoming these
social consequences of infertility is to marry another, usually
younger, woman, who has a child for you. For the Kuria,
and for the Zulu of South Africa, a close male relative of the
husband is chosen by the wife to have sexual relations with
her bride, and the resulting offspring become the recognized
children of the barren couple, not the biological parents.
For the Kikuyu, the biological father may be a villager or
someone chosen by either wife, or even, although rarely, the
male husband of one of the wives.

The marriage practice is so enshrined in Kikuyu culture
that the words for 'woman to woman marriage' and 'man
to woman marriage' are the same: *kuhikania* (the process of

getting married) and *uhiki* (the ceremony), with no difference in locally recognized rights for the partners in each case.[40]But the marriages could, and still do, bring their own castigation and difficulties. Regarded by local Christian churches as evil practices, some wives in same-sex marriages find themselves banned from religious community groups, unable to benefit from charitable donations and emotional support. In 1983 a Kenyan court case between two married women lasted more than a year, when Peris Nyakerario sued her wife, Agatha Kerubo, for breach of contract, because Mrs Kerubo threw her out of their marital home when the village priest no longer agreed to give her communion following their traditional wedding.[41]

Woman to woman marriages may happen as a sole marriage or as an additional marriage, so a heterosexual married couple can increase their family by the woman marrying another woman. In this case the new wife is not always brought into the house because the first woman cannot have children, and in one reported instance a first, heterosexual marriage produced several children. When the wife married again, this time to a woman, the new wife cared for the children of the original marriage.

The women were as varied in their circumstances as they were in their reasons for taking a woman as a wife. Mbura, a Kikuyu widow of more than forty years, told of a longing and a loss that resonated with me, although the arrangement was far from my own experience: 'I married Nimu because I could never have children myself. I did not even give birth to children who later died, nor did I experience any miscarriage. I remained the way I came out of my mother's womb. And now I'm getting old and there is no way I can

sit, think and decide to have a baby, because my time is over
. . . I think a lot about how my husband left me and how I
can't have a baby. That is why a cry of a baby makes me
happy and sad at the same time . . . So when I think about all
these things: how I can't have a child, how my husband died
and left me nothing, and how I have this illness, I ask Ngai
wenda mdathima na mutumia ungi (God bless me with another
woman). Won't you please send that woman here to my
home? Who knows, that woman might . . . give me a child
. . . Don't you see when I die I will be satisfied that I have left
somebody in that home, who shall continue and revive that
home?'[42]

I experienced such familiarity and empathy when I read
this because it is not only the want of a child that moves
Mbura, but a feeling that with her death comes the end of
all she has been: 'If I were to die as we speak, that would be
the end of it. I would be completely forgotten. No one would
ever mention my name. That is simply because there would
be no one to carry my name.'[43]

The childless often feel they will be forgotten, that the
memory of who we are and who our family has been is
an unbroken thread of procreation that will now end in
nothingness. It's not really true, of course; it is not only our
children who may carry memory of what we have done,
or of who we are, and for those of us fortunate enough to
have been born at a time and place where we can write
books, hold political office, work in medicine or any one of
a hundred such callings, we leave a professional testament
too. But it really is about luck. My grandmother was the first
of my maternal family to be literate; my ancestral family
were amongst the poorest people in the country. Had I been

born in India today, it's unlikely I'd have had any of the opportunities I've had. For some, even for many, involuntary childlessness brings not only an end to social inclusion and hope for a better future but the end of the memory of you.

But, unlike the Indian women who felt cast out and disgraced by many in their community, isolated by an un-alterable state, there were, among the African accounts, examples that showed collaboration between groups of women, not just the couples who entered into the same-sex marriages. One Kikuyu woman, Nduta, described as 'about ninety years old', had been married, had had three sons, who were all murdered by people in her husband's clan, anxious to steal their land; Nduta's mother-in-law then urged her to marry again, and this time to take a woman as her wife: 'When a woman is left alone, she should not be frightened, but must be brave. You must make yourself a queen, other-wise be a coward and everything you stand for will be taken away from you by those who are hungry for what you have . . . If you were a woman, and you had properties, you will be the first one to be stolen from by the men who thought they were more important than women . . . I lost many of them [properties] because I was a woman and had no sons. So my mother-in-law advised me to marry my own woman . . .'[44]

And there was also another, deeply affecting reason behind Nduta's marriage; she dreamt that her long-dead sons, poisoned in their youth, came to her, to thank her for taking Ciru as a wife: 'Thank you, Mother, for marrying Ciru for us. We are very grateful for bringing us dead people back home again. We are grateful indeed for we will always be watching over you. Nothing will ever harm you. We will take care of you. And then I would say, If I didn't marry Ciru for them, who else could I have married her for?' [45]

Some Kikuyu believe that when someone dies unexpectedly, tragically, too young, the life that they might have lived can still happen, that they will fulfil their chances through someone else. Nduta had married Ciru, as her sons might have done, thus keeping their former home as somewhere they continued to belong.[46] It was not only to honour them, but to live a life they might have lived. In similar fashion, the language of the Kuria reflects an imaginary or dead child as party to the relationship. These marriages are known as *mokamööna*, 'daughter-in-law marriage', carrying the idea of a younger woman marrying a female husband's dead or unborn son and becoming both daughter-in-law and wife in her new marriage.[47]

But while Nduta's way of living for her children was culturally marked, she was not unusual in seeing her dead sons in her sleep. Dead children and their voices often haunt the dreams of the childless parents they leave behind.

A Short Note on Perspective

One result of my own childlessness is that I see it as conse-
quential in stories that I encounter in a way that is not always
apparent to others. It makes me ponder my own perception
of other people's lives. Has childlessness become a tinted
glass through which I relate to humankind?

Despite improvements in recent years, Sri Lanka still has
a high degree of rural poverty. Even before the tsunami in
2004, it was estimated that five million people were living
on less than $12 a month, with a further three million
living on less than $15 a month. Support is based on the
family unit, so it is only by pooling resources and, in old
age, relying on sons and daughters, that the poor are able
to subsist. Poverty itself is undoubtedly the root cause of the
problems the people face, but to me, childlessness is a major
exacerbating factor

On the outskirts of Kandy and in Colombo I met men
and women without children. If illness or injury prevented
them from working, their hardship was extreme. Homeless
and without recourse to any financial aid, their survival
depended on the kindness of Buddhist monks or on a handful
of rupees begged from passers-by. It was difficult to imagine
what possible change of circumstance might alleviate their
difficulties.

At the end of a research trip to Sri Lanka, my husband

and I stayed in the Kandalama Hotel in Sigiriya. The hotel is surrounded by jungle. The eco-friendly design, by the celebrated architect Geoffrey Bawa, makes it looks as if it is becoming subsumed by vegetation and the jungle, with its coiling lush foliage and chattering, mischievous monkeys, is slowly encroaching on the civilization the hotel represents. We went on an accompanied walk, culminating in a visit to an old house in what had once been the village. It had been a thriving, bustling place, but, with the much-needed extension of the reservoir, the villagers had been relocated and now only a solitary man remains.

Dissanayake Mudiyanselage Gunurathne lives in a traditional house, with a vegetable garden and running water, although he proudly indicated the well that he had used for years. He never attended school. Suffering from polio when he was six, at the age of twelve he had an accident 'where his hip bone came out'. His working life was blighted by his continued health issues; he trained in sewing, made funeral uniforms for dressing the dead, but after another accident wasn't able to work the paddle. He never married – his disability and employment difficulties did not make him a good prospect. Gunurathne's background was one of abject poverty. Without work, only subsistence-level living was achievable; without children to care for him and support him in old age, even that would cease to be possible in later years.

He turned to making bowls from coconut shells for long hours each evening, and sold them at the local market. But when demand for the bowls dwindled, Gunurathne called one of the biggest employers in the area. Was the local hotel able to find him any work that his disability would not prevent him undertaking?

No one had lived in the old village, close to the hotel, since 1949, but what remained did offer a glimpse of life in an earlier time and Gunurathne was invited to live there. His house is in a small clearing off an overgrown path, close to where we found a large water monitor inexplicably halfway up a tree. The house is better equipped and presented than many others we had seen. The hotel ran a pipeline to the house to provide water and there is a garden where Gunurathne grows fruit and vegetables, and where his biggest worry was thirsty elephants, he told us, indicating the scattered remnants of the firecrackers that he used to frighten them. Tourists to the hotel come to see his house, and he welcomes them, showing the coconut shells he once again makes into pots to sell for a few coins.

In his new home his extended family frequently visit him, something they had done only rarely before; his nephews and nieces love to stay in the house that is part of their history. Gunurathne calls himself 'a very lucky man' and recalls his new beginning at the Kandalama Hotel on 25 June 2003 as his 'first day at Kandalama Hotel the glorious'.

Gunurathne's story is one of triumphing over poverty and hardship, of an unusual collaboration, worthy of emulation. But, for me, it is also about an unusual way of finding an independent means of living when you are childless and society assumes that the children you could never have will look after you when you are infirm or old. Yet perhaps my interpretation is a personal one, and the childlessness I see colouring his narrative with an indelible stain is only a reflection of my own.

A Short Note on Waiting

Waiting is a characteristic of childlessness for many people, as it was for me. There were the months of waiting, only to be disappointed by the pain and blood that marked each failure, the tortuous waiting for the hospital appointment that disclosed the problem and the unlikeliness of pregnancy, waiting for endless results, waiting for someone to say your childlessness is temporary. That was a halfway place to be – not childless, because to assume that title was to admit defeat, but also not a mother, not pregnant – a parent in waiting. I hated the indeterminacy, but only if it could be resolved in the way I wished it to be.

I grew up in a nowhere, nothing kind of place, not city or country, but my parents made the best of it and at weekends I was taken on long walks down old farm roads just ten minutes from our council estate, past cattle, sheep and even an old horse that one of the farmers kept as a pet for his children. Other Saturday afternoons we'd head to Glasgow and, if I was well behaved, I'd get a knickerbocker glory in the cafe of a department store on Argyll Street before we caught the train back home again. I did not quite belong in either the city or the countryside. In the Highlands I was, understandably, regarded as a townie, yet when I first moved to London, the crowds, the sheer volume of people, made me fearful and ill at ease.

And so it was with waiting. I did not belong with mothers or expectant women, but I did not feel I could reconcile myself to joining the childless either. Even after an early menopause, when I knew there was no possibility of children at all, I felt ill at ease in childlessness support groups, was impatient to move on and to negotiate my own path through the rest of my life, rather than be cossetted in sympathy.

This sense of exclusion had its own effects. It made me want to explore as many ways of being childless as I could. People who had lost only children wrote to me, in response to a call for anyone who would share their bereavement, and several mentioned their feeling of not belonging. They had no living child, but they were parents all the same. These grieving parents did not feel welcome at support groups for the childless. One woman wrote that she felt she had to spend the whole meeting apologising because she had once had a daughter. She told me she had only gone to see how other people coped in this new world she was trying to navigate, but instead had found that her parenthood excluded her, just as her grief set her apart from those whose children were still living.

Time passes. I have grown accustomed to London – it's even a home of sorts now. I've adapted to my childlessness too. My life has adapted to accommodate its uneasy inevitability. I am not waiting any more.

5

Those Who are Childless Parents

In June 2009 Kazumi and Neil Puttick brought their only child, five-year-old Sam, from the hospital so he could die at home. The following Sunday they drove from Wiltshire to Beachy Head in Sussex, a trip of 150 miles. When they stepped off the high chalky clifftop they carried the body of their child in a rucksack.

The Putticks chose to take their own lives rather than face a future as childless parents. For those parents who try to navigate the minutes, hours, days and months that follow their bereavement, the world too often seems like a hostile place.

The childless parents I spoke to all agreed that theirs was a position of exclusion. It didn't seem to matter where in the world they were from or where they lived, or how old their son or daughter was they died; the fundamental understanding of their own self was distorted or lost altogether, and their society did not seem to have a place for them. They often felt excluded from discussions of childlessness and from the activities and responsibilities and pure joys of parenting. They were proud of their maternal or paternal role – still mothers and fathers, in the same way that I am my father's daughter even though my dad is now dead – but also anxious for support in navigating this world they now found themselves in. Finding a life for themselves was about resolution, marrying the permanence of their status as parents with the crisis of the loss of a child.[1]

Those Who are Stillbirth Parents

For one group of childless parents, those whose child is still-born, there is yet another facet to these feelings of margin-alization. It has only been in recent times that the parents of stillborn children are allowed to confront their loss and mourn their child. As recently as the 1980s, the mother of a stillborn baby would be given no contact with her dead child; its body would be quickly taken away and buried, often in a common municipal grave, while the mother was still drugged and recovering from the birth.[2]

In an interview for the *Telegraph*, Sheena Byrom, a midwife of thirty years, recalled: 'There was a blanket of silence over stillbirth. I remember feeling desperately upset for the mothers, but we were discouraged from talking to them about it because the view was that we would upset them.'[3]

The *Journal of Family Nursing* considers case studies from the period when stillbirth was seen as something to avoid discussing, often with the well-meaning intention of pro-tecting the mother from further pain. The individual experiences show the psychological harm that could result, and the paper stresses the importance of today's caregiving support for the bereaved, specifically being invited to spend time with the dead baby and being supported by rituals of commemoration and burial.[4]

But not everyone agrees that the new recommendations,

which encourage the mother to hold her dead child and perhaps create a memory box with foot or hand prints or photographs, are better. Dr Patricia Hughes, Professor of Psychiatry at the University of London, carried out a study which surprisingly showed that mothers who held their stillborn baby were more likely to suffer depression during any subsequent pregnancy. Furthermore, they had more problems bonding with children born afterwards.[5] But, significantly, the study did not explore the benefits or otherwise for those who did not have any other children.

Ellen Smith is forty and lives in Manchester.[6] Five years ago, in the eighth month of her pregnancy, she was told that her daughter, Megan, did not have a heartbeat. Megan was to be the only child of Ellen and her husband Ed; a medically necessary hysterectomy in 2014 means that they can have no more children. Following the news of Megan's condition, Ellen was given an emergency caesarean. 'They were very good at the hospital. They brought her to me and I sat up in bed, holding her. All I could feel was a great rush of love. This was my little girl.'

Ellen and Ed took photos of each other holding her and had them framed. 'One nurse offered to take pictures of us altogether, so we have that too. She was so tiny, but so very perfect. It was heartbreaking, of course, but there was also a lot of love. We'd had a lot of attempts and it was the first time we had got this far. I thought, I'm a mother now. A grieving mother, but still.'

They had a small family funeral and buried Megan in a plot where they will be buried when their time comes. They both agreed that the most difficult time was when the ceremony was over. Ed said his biggest problem was in the office where he works. 'This will sound really bad. But if we had had a toddler or an older child and it had died, I know everyone would have been supportive. There would have been bereavement leave and kindness. But a lot of people – well, a lot of men, it's really only men in our office – seemed to think that because Megan was stillborn it was different and that it would all be back to business as usual as soon as arrangements were made and Ellen was out of the hospital. No one ever said anything directly, but after a couple of months I could really sense that people didn't see it as such a big deal. But she was our daughter.'

Ellen found that 'People were more sympathetic to me, at first anyway. But there was a lot of those "she's in a better place" platitudes and at least one good friend told me outright she thought naming a dead baby was morbid.' For her, the worst part of her experience was that her grief was heightened by guilt. Despite medical reassurance that there was nothing she could have done to prevent the heart failure, she continually questioned her actions during the pregnancy and wondered if she could have done something to save Megan.

Ellen and Ed's experience is not uncommon. Many women experience shame or guilt at stillbirth, and the attitudes of those around the parents can be surprising. *ABC News* carried an account of grandparents who were 'horrified' that their daughter wanted to name her stillborn child.[7] In June 2015 the *New York Times* published a piece called 'Stillbirth: Your Stories'. It is prefaced by an interview with Dr Eleni Michailidis, who discusses the loss of her own son and ends by stressing the way that people often don't speak about stillbirth, because it's too upsetting or because people just don't want to hear about it. The article is a catalogue of ninety-seven accounts by women who have experienced stillbirths. Many commemorate their lost child, others speak because they are tired of being silenced. Yet it was not the lack of acknowledgement of their bereavement alone that hurt and surprised Eleni: 'I was a mother. All my hormones were telling me that and the waves of love. Yet within a year I just went back to being someone without children. Maybe what I wanted most was someone to say I'd been a mum.'

Those Who are the Bereaved

Many childless parents report that all of their thoughts are divided into before and afterwards. Before loss, they are sure of their identity; afterwards, they miss not only their beloved son or daughter but the place in the world that they believed the parental relationship afforded them. Time itself becomes unreliable, because its passage is no longer reflected in the growth and development of a child. These strange and bewildering perceptions of time in the period following the loss of a child add to the feeling of detachment from the rest of society.

Dr Adi Barak from the University of Chicago and Dr Ronit Leichtentritt from Tel Aviv University have researched the perception of time in the narrative of bereaved parents.[8] They identify different narrative possibilities. Time may appear to stop altogether, because human time has stopped for their child – because it is no longer relevant for the son or daughter, it is no longer relevant for the parent. Yossi Zur lost his son in a suicide terrorist attack and wrote this poem:

Blondi, my kid
You are just a kid
Almost seventeen
And in this age you'll stay
For an eternity[9]

For one mother, it meant the continuing rearrangement of the clothes in her daughter's closet in accordance with the seasons; an attempt to 'insert a dimension of time advancement for the daughter who had stopped advancing in time'.[10]

Other parents become fixated on the inevitability of time passing, no matter how much they wish they could stop it. They may be preoccupied by thoughts of the material changes to their child's body, but also of a more spiritual transformation, seeing their offspring as having had an experience that is beyond their own. One father imagined his son as a father-like figure who encouraged him to get over his loss and move on with his life.[11] These odd perceptions of time only add to the feeling of being apart from society, made other by loss.

Phil is from the west coast of America.[12] His son was a boy called Joe. Joe's mother had died in childbirth and so this son was not only a precious loved child in his own right, but also the last cherished, biological link with Phil's late wife. 'He looked like her – his hair, the tight curls, the brown eyes – and every year that we had together was like a year gifted back from her dying.'

There were fifteen such years, but then one night a drunk driver swerved off the road and hit Joe as he was coming home from a friend's house. He died instantly. Phil tells me that this is the smallest of comforts, but comfort it is, in a place where there is none else to be found. 'Everyone is kind, everyone tries to be sympathetic, but suddenly there's an end to all of the things that made up your day, your week, your year. For six months after, I still watched the school baseball team every time they had a game, because the alternative, not to go at all, seemed so much worse. There're no parent-teacher meetings, no plans for college, no Sunday drives out to the park. The world of parenting that made up who I was outside of my professional life was gone, suddenly and irrevocably. I didn't belong any more, but I was still Joe's dad, and that was the hardest thing of all.'

Phil reflected that Joe's lack of siblings meant he did not have the motivation he observed in other bereaved parents in the support groups he occasionally attended. They were pushed back into some kind of normalcy by a desire to protect and raise their other children. For Phil, the activities relating to child-rearing would never again have the same significance, the same relevance, both in his own and in others' eyes. He described himself as being relegated to the position of an 'odd, solitary figure'. He had become a lone, childless man, watching children, often regarded with suspicion because he was outside of the sphere of family, accepted and understood only by those who knew of the loss of his son.

Alma was in her forties and had lost her infant daughter, Melanie, when she was a teenager.[13] 'I didn't love her dad,' she told me, 'was barely a child myself, but I loved that little girl with all my heart. I was so determined to be a better mother than mine had been, and to be everything to her.' Melanie died of sudden infant death syndrome. 'It was twenty-seven years ago and I still remember every second of that night somehow. I still feel like a mum too, because I know I had all the days before it and that she was mine.'

For Alma, her dead daughter is still part of her life, made real by her imagination. 'Even now, it's difficult if someone asks if I have children. I'm childless as far as society is concerned. But I still speak to my daughter every day. In my imagination, my daughter is someone I can share my experience with now. In my twenties and thirties, like all women, I had people ask me when I was going to start having a family, and I kept wanting to say I won't be starting, I already had one, but somehow the words never quite came out. I feel I don't belong somehow. I'm a nursery nurse and at one of my first job interviews they asked if I felt not having kids of my own might make me not the best person for the job. I did tell them about Melanie, although after I was angry with myself and thought I should have said, it doesn't matter, because it doesn't really, but I wanted to talk about Melanie to them, wanted to feel that the experience of her was helping me, even if it had all ended. It's still me, still who I am, I was a mum – do I ever stop being one?'

Alma was so young when she bore and lost her daughter that her child has somehow grown with her after death, giving her a way to manage her loss. Time passes and the daughter of her imagination continues to grow and develop, shaped by her mother's life experience.

Dr Kay Talbot, herself a bereaved mother, researches mothers coming to terms with the death of an only child.[14] She emphasizes 'the search for meaningful ways to continue "mothering" as part of a new, more integrated identity which acknowledges the child's death but also preserves the child's memory and honours the woman's past life as a mother'.[15]

Those Who are Missing Children

When a child dies, the absoluteness of the parent's loss offers some closure. But this does not help the bereaved to navigate the company of childless adults, a group which they now found themselves unwillingly part of. Missing children – abducted, taken or lost during political upheaval and revolution – offer a different perspective on childless parents because of the thin threads of fragile hope that keep them connected to their offspring until their own death. For these men and women, the only true understanding is found in the company of others in the same position, both as a means to find out what has happened but also to achieve redress as a committed group.

The civil war in Sri Lanka finally ended in May 2009, but more than two years later 630 children were still missing. Reports cited by UNICEF claimed that 64 per cent of those missing had been child soldiers of the now defeated Liberation Tigers of Tamil Eelam (LTTE). In the last phase of the war, more than 300,000 civilians were displaced, corralled into ever-shrinking areas, while the government troops advanced on them. By the time they arrived in the camps, many parents were distraught, without any idea of the whereabouts of their offspring.

In Sri Lanka I met the activist Visaka Dharmadasa.[16] Her own twenty-one-year-old son went missing after Tamil Tigers attacked his military base in Kilonochchi. Her son had no identification tag: 'The army didn't think it was important! If he had been wearing an ID tag, I would have known what happened to him.'

Visaka is the founder of two organizations: the Association

of War Affected Women (AWAW), for mothers of missing children, regardless of what side of the conflict they were on; and the Association of Parents of Servicemen Missing in Action (PSMIA). AWAW was only established after Visaka had interacted with Tamil mothers and realized the commonality of suffering. Women who had lost husbands or children or both were involved, and their aim was to bring the two communities together. Visaka's work now focuses on peace-building. So far, because of her determined campaigning, changes have been executed, including the issuing of identity cards to all soldiers, and the implementation of training schemes to encourage women to become effective leaders and advocates for peace. 'It's not just my work. I was pushed in this situation and I know, in order to save the children of my country, I have to do this.'

Visaka's house in Kandy is both elegant and cosy, with ebony furniture, wide windows, and a welcoming bowl of bananas brought in from the garden to offer to us. I asked her about her son, if it was worse not knowing what had happened to him. She replied, 'Not knowing means there's hope, still hope.'

Visaka recounted the story of Marla Mariani, a grandmother and founder of the human rights' organization Grandmothers of the Plaza De Mayo, which tries to reunite family members lost and separated during the Argentinian dictatorship between 1976 and 1983. Mariani finally found her granddaughter after thirty-nine years of searching. In Sri Lanka, a country of contradictions, of sparkling seas, dense jungles, elephants, tsunamis, poverty and precious stones, Visaka's hope and my imagination saw a series of tunnels, of dark hidden places where boys and girls, held captive since the war, waited still for reunification.

In her book *Circle of Love Over Death*, Matilde Mellibovsky gathered together accounts of the mothers whose children had been taken or had disappeared in Argentina. Mellibovsky's own daughter, Graciela, was abducted on 25 September 1976. 'A disappearance places you in a very large, dense cloud from which you cannot escape, because in the unconscious a hope always survives, while you rationally assume the absoluteness of death,' she writes. 'When we deal with one of the disappeared, an unknown, culturally uncharted relationship is established. The disappeared person himself agonizes in his impotence, with the conviction that his life will be totally erased from the face of the earth, that nobody else will know about him. In the same way, his mother lives out the agony of uncertainty; she cannot prevent her thoughts from accompanying the disappeared at all times: in the darkness, in the hunger, sickness, torture, in his call for his mother, in the filth, and in the humiliation; and in the death, in the decomposition of his well-loved matter, in the rotting of his bones . . . When someone disappears by force, everything remains surrounded with a tangle of conjectures, indeterminacies, doubts.'[17]

Both of Ilda Irrustita De Micucci's children were abducted from their home in Buenos Aires on 11 November 1976. A group of men arrived at her house in the small hours of the morning, looking for her son, Daniel. But he had already left for work, and so they took her daughter, ostensibly just to interrogate her. Ilda and her husband travelled to Pilar to warn Daniel what had happened but, by the time they got there, the men were already collecting her son. They detained the whole family then, in separate cars, with hoods covering their heads so they had no idea where they were going. But when Ida and her husband, Pepe, were released the following night on the Pan-American highway, their children were not. They never saw them again.

Pepe was a member of the armed forces, a career that defined who he was. When he and his wife tried to join in solidarity with other parents whose children were missing, he found himself surrounded by people who were filled with hatred for the military. Ilda explained: 'He really became divided into two parts, one part the father who lost his children and had to do the impossible to recover them, and the other part formed by his military background . . . You know, he died without having gotten any news about his children. Actually, we never got any news. But nevertheless, I remained eager to fight in whatever way I could, to do whatever was feasible, because I could not imagine then (or even now) that they would never reappear.'[18]

In the United States FBI statistics suggest that almost half a million children go missing there every year, while figures from the organization Missing Kids UK show that a child goes missing every three minutes in Britain. The term 'ambiguous loss' was coined by Professor Pauline Boss from the University of Minnesota to encapsulate the experience of those whose loved one is missing.[19] The sufferer does not know if their loss will have closure and therefore how to progress with their own life. Instead they live with 'frozen grief', unable to find comfort in the rituals that mark someone's passing, vacillating between hopefulness and mourning.[20]

Tiffany Sessions was last seen in February1989. The FBI

claim that the search to find her has been the biggest ever in the state of Florida, but, despite detaining numerous suspects, her current state remains unknown. Tiffany was twenty-one, an only child and a student at Florida State University. In the aftermath of her disappearance, her mother, Hilary, wrote a book about trying to come to terms with not knowing. When Tiffany had been missing for eighteen years, the National Centre for Missing and Exploited Children (NCMEC) agreed to take on her case and, as part of their search, created an age-enhanced photo of what Tiffany might look like at the age of thirty-nine. Her mother hesitated to open it: 'Whatever the enhancement looked like, it would permanently change the last known photo of my baby. Will I recognize her? Will she still look like my little girl? I'm not sure I want to open the file, I'm scared, it's been so long. When I did, I looked at every feature, from the eyebrows, the creases around her eyes, her smile, and her hair, to see if I would recognize my baby when I saw her.'[21]

Glenn Miller, supervisor of the Forensic Imaging Unit at NCMEC, described the limitations of the process for *New Scientist*: 'Artificially ageing the face of a child is very difficult because children's faces grow and change rapidly.' Yet parents of dead children are also seeking age-enhancement photos to see what their children would have looked like had they still been alive. Pat Frankish is a clinical psychologist who researches parents' reaction to the death of a child. She does not regard the current interest in age-enhancement images of dead children as being in the parents' best interest. 'It seems to me that the age progression of a dead child is a denial of the fact they have gone. It's a refusal to move on with life. These parents may be shutting themselves off from the experience of living in the present. We don't age-progress adults who die early into old age. But when a child dies you also grieve for this sense of unlimited possibility.'[22]

Yet for parents suffering from ambiguous loss, it's a way of imagining their child in the present, of feeling connected to them despite the passing of time, as well as a tool to help find them. Just as Melanie's dead child had continued to grow in her imagination, so the parents of the missing try to fill the years of their loss with a sense of who their child has become. It is a way both of preserving hope and also of preparing for reunion.

Those Who are the Parents of Stolen Children

In Australia from 1910 to 1970, between 10 and 33 per cent of all Aboriginal children were removed from their parental homes as part of a process of assimilation. Based on the assumption that white people were superior to native Australians, these stolen children were placed with white families and taught to reject their indigenous culture. In some cases, they were informed that their parents had disowned them or were not fit to care for them. *Bringing Them Home*, the 1997 report of the National Inquiry into the Separation of Aboriginal and Torres Strait Islander Children from Their Families, notes that these abductions were often as brutal as snatching the child while parents were away or even from the mother's arms. But there were other threatening ways of removing children. In one instance, in Gippsland in south-eastern Australia, a young woman who was pregnant, aged fourteen, was approached by a welfare-board officer, who said that, as the child was fatherless and illegitimate, they would like to place it in a home with a white family. After the birth the girl was reunited with the baby's father, whom she married. When she was asked to sign the papers for adoption, she refused, saying she had changed her mind. The officer replied, 'If you change your mind and you renege on this particular deal, I'm going to have you charged with having carnal knowledge under the age of fourteen.' She acquiesced to the adoption under the threat of prosecution and her child was taken.[23]

In perhaps the most sinister machinations of all, a child might be reported as already dead: 'A mother [single teenager] had a child in a home, and went out to provide some sort of basis for rearing the child. The child was left there, and when the mother came back, they told her that the child had died. And twenty-five years later we have a request from a person to find his mother, and we approached the mother, and she now has gone through the grieving of the person dying and now coming to terms with his resurrection.'[24]

Understandably much has been written about the experience of these children, taken from their families and culture, and raised in an alien one. But what of the parents who were left behind, unknowing and unable to contact their sons and daughters? The report found it difficult to identify women who were prepared to speak of their experience, for the most part because, no matter how helpless they had been at the time, they still felt guilty that they had allowed their child to be taken. 'We end up feeling helpless in front of our mother's pain. We see how hurt they have been. We see that they judge themselves harshly, never forgiving themselves for losing their children – no matter that they were part of ongoing systematic removal of Aboriginal children.'[25]

Fathers too felt the emotional burden of being unable to hold their families together. 'Mum was kidnapped. My grandfather was away working at the time, and he came home and found that his kids had been taken away, and he didn't know nothing about it. Four years later he died of a broken heart. He had a breakdown and was sent to Kew [Psychiatric] Hospital. He was buried in a pauper's grave and on his death certificate he died of malnutrition, ulcers and plus he had bedsores. He was fifty-one.'[26] The loss of their children was compounded by factors such as racism and discrimination, and the sense that, within the extended community, they no longer had one of the most valuable roles, that of parent, and indeed had been found unfit for that role.

Bringing Them Home called for an apology by the Australian parliament, which heralded the first annual National Sorry Day on 28 May 1998. Ten years later, on 13 February 2008 the prime minister, Kevin Rudd, did issue an apology to the 'Stolen Generations'. He also called on 'the determination of all Australians, Indigenous and non-Indigenous, to close the gap that lies between us in life expectancy, educational achievement and economic opportunity'.[27] A policy commission was set up and the prime minister's report, *Closing the Gap*, is published every year. But by 2016 only two of the seven objectives had been met, and there is no tracking of the number of children still being forcibly taken and put into care.

Investigative journalism by John Pilger suggested that the problem is more widespread now than it has ever been. As of June 2013, 14,000 Aboriginal children had been removed from their families, five times the number that had been stolen in 1997, when the National Inquiry report was written. In 2012 the co-ordinator general for the Northern Territory was sacked when she revealed that £44 million was spent on removing Aboriginal children, in contrast to the £275,000 spent on supporting indigenous, poor families.[28]

In 2014 the organization Grandmothers Against Removals (GAR) was founded by Aunty Hazel Collins. Its principal aim is to reduce the number of indigenous children being taken from their families and put into care, but it also works to reunite those who have been separated. Crucially, it campaigns for a proper implementation of the recommendations in *Bringing Them Home*. Laura Wradjiri of GAR told me: 'When they first started taking children in the 1950s and 1960s there were 2,800 in care. Now we're in 2017 and there are 18,622, and a third of them are Aboriginal children. Yet we only make up 2.2 per cent of the country. I had my three children removed. When they take the children, they don't give them back. There were fifty-four recommendations of the report – and they weren't implemented. One lady, she had eight children and they took all eight, split them up like.'[29]

Laura accepts that the indigenous people may need more support with their families, but she argues that the huge amount of money spent on taking children and raising them in institutions would be better spent on the communities themselves: 'The Stolen Generation hasn't stopped. There's a second stolen generation. I'd like to see the support being built up around families and communities, for them to work with the families. The system is meant to meet children's needs. They have an obligation to make sure every child is safe. But it isn't working. They're failing.'

Laura's tribe is matriarchal; their support clinic is named Werribee, a word that means 'backbone', which refers to the backbone of all the female ancestors that have gone before. The role of the women in her tribe is not only mothering but passing on the child's heritage, something which Laura clearly identifies as under threat from a predominately patriarchal state: 'If you don't have your culture, you don't have self-identity. If you don't [have it], you're lost. It's our purpose. We have a very unique method of raising children. You've got the extended family and the community. We have cultural responsibility.'

In taking children from their communities, Laura feels indigenous peoples are denied both their role as parent and the ability to fulfil their responsibility to educate the child in his or her native culture and language: 'When the colonizers came here, it was forbidden for us to speak our language. But I still know some words. We pass it down, and what words I know I teach my family. When the children are removed from their own society, they don't learn our ways or the words . . . It's not just here either. I'm in touch with indigenous women in North America. It's happening there to them too.'[30]

Research from the University of Queensland adds support to Laura's understanding of her experience. It shows that there is considerable over-representation of indigenous children in care and points out that the situation is very similar to that of other native peoples in Canada, the United States and New Zealand.[31] Interviews with lawyers who were involved with indigenous communities in child protection

allowed researchers to explore the processes and legal structures that are being implemented. Their conclusion was not
that children must never be removed from indigenous parents, because on occasion circumstances might necessitate
this, but that aspects of child protection could be improved
to reduce the need for removal.[32] There also needed to be a
greater commitment to reunification; one lawyer reported
that staff saw themselves more as 'watchdogs', keeping children away from what they perceived as harmful indigenous
communities.[33]

The Stolen Generation is a perpetuating cycle that can
only be broken by 'a more participatory and inclusive frame-
work that strongly involves indigenous people in the issues
that directly affect them'.[34] Creative solutions are needed, a
'community and collective response' that allows children to
grow up within their communities, but also allows parents
to carry on the responsibility of cultural transmission.[35]
The childless indigenous parent loses not only their son or
daughter but, from their perspective, the chance to actively
participate in the continuation of their diminishing and
threatened cultures. Time passing without their child denies
them the ability to watch his or her growth and development,
and hastens a decline in the fabric of the society that made
them who they are. It is a double loss of identity, one immediate, the other more subtle and redolent of decay.

In 1969, in Warwickshire, UK, a hospital chaplain and a
small group of bereaved parents came together, because of
the lack of recognition of their particular kind of experience,
to form an organization known as The Compassionate
Friends.[36] It now has a special forum for those who have no

surviving children. Its aim is to bring together those who have suffered this particular kind of grief and its repercussions.

A pamphlet, *Childless Parents*, offers advice and tells of shared experience, but one passage caught my attention above all.[37] Entitled 'Other People', it warns of the thoughtless questions that may be asked, such as, 'Why did you have only one child?' or the hints that 'You can always have more children, even adopt'. Throughout the summary of experiences, the feeling of isolation, of difference, prevails. There are the difficulties of communicating with those who have children and want to speak about them, and of trying to identify with the childless or child-free; all are exacerbated by bewilderment at the person you now find yourself to be.

As I read the booklet I think how it could easily have been written to support someone who is infertile or childless by circumstance. The only difference is that the childless parents are grieving for a person they have loved and for an identity they once had, not for one who will never be born and for a person they will never be.

Sally and Neil Holland lost their fourteen-year-old son Luke. While Sally finds the term 'childless parents' apt for their circumstances, she feels that language itself excludes them. There is no term in English for who they have become: 'If you lose your parents you're an orphan; if you lose your husband you're a widow and if you lose your wife you're a widower. But there's no word for losing your child. It's as though it's so terrible they couldn't even give it a name.'[38]

A Short Note on Josh

In the midst of writing we receive terrible news, Al's dearest friend, the best man at our wedding, has a teenage son who is dying of a brain tumour.

Debbie and Tony only have one child and so, inevitably, when the last trial fails to happen because Josh's condition has deteriorated so quickly, too soon, we find ourselves waiting for dear, kind, good people to become childless parents.

We learn the news through Facebook. Debbie and Tony, like my husband, Alan, grew up in New Zealand, but now they live in Colorado. Before that they lived in Florida. There is a web of people who care stretched across three continents, two states, many countries, and social media, for all the bad press it gets, is a great way of letting everyone know what is happening. The updates, however, show me a glimpse of something that I have missed, for all of my listening, for all of my trying. One of Debbie's friend's posts:

'Many years ago, a group of women joined a moms' group when our children were babies or little. We spent a lot of time together, including play dates, GNOs, bunko nights, lunches, field trips and outings, beach trips, Disney, family milestones, baby showers, birthday parties, house moves, scavenger hunts, dance recitals, and just hanging out and much much more. We supported each other through ups and downs and the woes of motherhood. And even though some of us have moved away, we still keep in touch and give our love and support.'

I had an image then that stays with me even now, of the preparation for adulthood that is so much part of having a child. I imagined all the first-date, first-job, study-or-not-study conversations, shared with other parents whose children grew up alongside yours. I remember my parents having them at school open days and over the garden fence, or in supermarket aisles when they bumped into someone unexpectedly. With Josh's death, all of those parenting plans will go too, will be no more than a ghost of a future, while the parenting experience of the past remains and continues to define the people that our friends become.

Towards the end, the act of departure seems so great that even Debbie confesses to Facebook that there are moments where being in the room is almost too hard for her.

She takes to counting the lack of breaths as she observes his body shutting down. The ending seems slow, drawn out, for those of us reading on a screen, but, as long as those breaths continue, I think, Tony and Debbie have a living child.

When Josh passes, on 14 March 2017, Debbie, raw and exhausted, posts that her heart is broken, although her son has found peace.

Fly, little boy, Fly.

Afterwards, in the weeks that follow, I see the unravelling of the life that she and Tony have had; I watch their careful construction of a childless one. It is so familiar from the mails and Skype conversations with strangers, all of the childless parents who have let me listen, but also different because we are not detached at all.

Debbie writes: 'We're working on breaking the habit of looking in to check up on Joshua every time we walk down the hall. We're slowly picking things up and putting them in his room as now we know he won't need them 'here' any more. I'm learning that I don't need to pick up certain things at the supermarket, and that the seats in the car can now stay back, not be moved forward so long legs can fit. Every day it's little things.'

And of course, those milestones keep coming. Saddest of all, perhaps, on Mother's Day she posts: 'So to those other Mothers I know that have lost their child and have, like me, become "unMothered" – enjoy a beautiful day filled with memories of a different sort. Remember the beautiful moments, the crazy ones, and the downright ugly ones – they made us who we are today.'

Unmothered. It is sad and apt, but I do not think she is unmothered. I do not think she ever can be. Those moments that she remembers are the memories of a parent. She will always be Josh's mother, even if he is no longer her living son.

A Short Note on Kahlo

Mexican artist Frida Kahlo was the victim of a horrific traffic accident that left her spinal cord broken when an iron handrail pierced her abdomen and uterus. She never successfully carried a child to term.

In 1932 Kahlo painted *Henry Ford Hospital*. Kahlo is shown lying alone on a hospital bed, flat on her back after the miscarriage that she had suffered. The 'little Diego', the son she had longed for, had not developed in her womb: 'the foetus did not form, for it came out all disintegrated'.[1] Six images float above her, connected by blood-red cords to her hand as it lies on her still-swollen belly. There is an orchid, a gift from her husband, Diego Rivera; something she described as 'the idea of a sexual thing mixed with the sentimental'; and a snail, which symbolizes the slowness of her miscarriage. There is a foetus, her unborn son, who has a strong resemblance to Diego; a pelvic bone; an anatomical representation of a female abdomen; and an autoclave, a medical receptacle used for sterilizing surgical instruments, which symbolizes both the procedure and the fact that Kahlo too was sterile.

Six things. A tear runs down her face.

Far in the background there are the outlines of the city of Detroit, where Diego is working on a mural. There is a desert between her and the buildings, an arid, barren landscape that separates her from her beloved. It is her own infertility too, her inability to give him a son, coming between her and Diego. In her diary, Kahlo wrote: 'Children are the days and here it is stopped.'[2]

The phrase catches me. I am moved for Kahlo, but also for myself, and for all of the others, with our betraying bodies. Kahlo had been pregnant before but had been compelled to have an abortion when the foetus's position in her fractured pelvis made the pregnancy untenable. The second time too, using castor oil and medication, she tried to push out the child she was told could never be born. When the abortion failed, she was given the hope that she might be able to carry the unborn baby till it was old enough to be delivered by Caesarean.

Less than two weeks after her miscarriage, in a letter to her physician, Dr Eloesser, she wrote: 'I have wanted to write to you for a long time than you can imagine. I had so looked forward to having a little Dieguito that I cried a lot, but it's over, there is nothing else that can be done except to bear it.'[3]

Two years later Diego finished the three-part mural *Epic of the Mexican People*. Frida Kahlo is depicted as one of the workers, as is her sister Cristina, whom Diego had recently taken as a lover, but his wife is obscured, set behind his lover and her two children. Kahlo did not paint for the rest of that year.

In 1945 Kahlo painted *Without Hope*. She turns to us, the viewers. Tears stream down her face as she looks out at us from a rocky desert landscape that represents her own failed fertility. From her mouth is a funnel and from it comes only death, carcases, rotting fish, a skull. It is as if these are what she sees coming out of her body – a grim, sickening alternative to the child she could never have.

6

Those Who Choose: Child-free

The childless by choice are a group as diverse as those who suffer from involuntary childlessness, but are more constrained by geography, with women in some cultures unable to identify with the concept at all. For example, a demographic study of recently married women in Vietnam failed to identify a single subject who did not wish to have children.[1] The reason for a woman's choice may also directly or indirectly affect how she is treated by society. Some who are child-free for religious reasons, for example, will enjoy respect, while those who simply did not wish to have offspring may meet with discrimination and questioning. Sometimes the prejudice is casual and unthinking, but at others it may be legislative, even sinister. And, of course, the nature and intensity of prejudice within a given society will vary according to gender and sexuality.

In the English-speaking world, the semantic appropriateness of the term 'childless' to describe those who have no wish to have children is contested. For many in that group, the word itself is wrong, emphasizing the lack of something that they never wanted in the first place, reinforcing negative societal stereotypes. Many prefer the term 'child-free', feeling that it is more positive, of equal status to those who have children. But it is by no means a universal preference.

The author Carolyn Morrell takes exception to the term 'child-free', noting that it has a 'presumptuous ring' to it, suggesting that women who are childless wish to be free of children and may somehow be antagonistic to them and are therefore (again) somehow inferior to mothers.[2]

National data do not generally particularize the reason for childlessness and this lack has been redressed by countless academic studies. It wasn't until the 1980s, however, that the language in these studies changed to specify those who were 'intentionally' or 'voluntarily' childless. By the 1990s this had morphed into 'child-free' and 'childless by choice'.[3]

Some facts about this group seem to contradict received wisdom. The common notion that childless women may not have had children for economic reasons, for example, belies the fact that, if you are a woman, the more you earn, or the more educated you are, the more likely you are to be childless. Surprisingly, there are no significant economic variables for men.[4] Research also discredits the notion that people who are child-free have chosen their career over having a family. Laura Scott, director of the Childless by Choice Project, interviewed 121 women and fifty men in North America about their reasons for opting for a child-free life.[5] From the eighteen options listed in the survey, the three most popular motives were:

> I love our life, our relationship, as it is, and having a child won't enhance it
> I value freedom and independence
> I do not want to take on the responsibility of raising a child.

These findings are borne out by an academic study in 2007 which found the most common reasons for being child-free were:

An aversion to the lifestyle changes that come with parenthood
Rejection of the maternal role
Selfishness and feeling either unsuited or proficient but unwilling to be a parent.[6]

Taking an overview, a recent article in the *Journal of Population Research* concluded that 'Contrary to popular stereotype only a minority of childless people forgo parenthood specifically to focus on their career.'[7]

The most marked difference between men's and women's decisions to be child-free is that women make the choice for altruistic reasons and are far more likely to stress that it is a joint agreement made with a partner, whereas men tend to focus on the consequences to their own daily lives and habits.[8]

Regardless of the reasons for choosing to be child-free, societal stigma exists, with studies demonstrating that parents of either gender are perceived as warmer than non-parents, while couples are viewed more favourably if they seem more likely to have children.[9]

The personal experience of the different groups, however, shows more variation than these findings might suggest, as well as, in some cases, commonality with those who are involuntarily childless. But the decision to be sexually active and not have children also depends on the availability of contraception, so even if you have made a choice to avoid

CHILDLESS VOICES

becoming a parent, some countries and cultures may not support that decision.

The World Health Organization reported in 2016 that globally 225 million people would like to be able to prevent pregnancy but did not use contraception. This is due to a wide range of factors, including extreme poverty, cultural and religious opposition, and restricted or limited access to birth control. In Papua New Guinea research suggests that men do not like their wives to use contraceptives, whereas regions such as Latin America, where access to birth control has historically been difficult, now have the fastest growth in contraceptive use in the world. Restricting contraceptive access is a way to control reproductive freedom and to increase dwindling populations, and may be enforced by governments. We saw in an early chapter how forced sterilization impacts on the lives of men and women, but restrictions and legislation designed to force procreation also exist. In 2014 143 of 231 members of the Iranian parliament voted to ban all sterilization operations, the second most popular form of contraception in the country, and prohibit any advertising of birth control.[10] Violation can carry the same punishment as abortion, up to five years in prison and a blood-money fine.[11] And in 2015 Radio Free Asia reported that North Korea had banned abortions and all contraception in an attempt to increase its rapidly diminishing population. For men and women in these circumstances, the alternatives to parenting are enforced celibacy, backstreet abortions or imprisonment.

Child-free: Heterosexual Men

In the 1950s an unmarried man was often assumed to be a homosexual. In current-day Western society this obviously isn't the case, but heterosexual men still report surprising attitudes to their choice not to embark on fatherhood. An Australian study using both male and female informants found that there was almost no difference between the negative perceptions of men and women. The fewer children you had, the less positively your personality was viewed, with the voluntarily childless being described as selfish, materialistic and career-focused.[12] An earlier study from the US indicated that while both men and women who were voluntarily childless were viewed negatively, women were perceived slightly more so.[13] This view was reflected in the experience of the British child-free I spoke to.

David, thirty-four, a lawyer from north London, has been married for eight years to Katy, a research chemist. Neither of them wants a family, but David recalls that around four years ago the gentle questions began. At first it was his parents, dropping frequent hints that they were getting on and would like to be young enough to enjoy their grandchildren. David found it odd that they assumed it was Katy's career that was making them delay, and he was quick to tell them that it was a mutual decision and that they valued their current lifestyle too much to change it. David didn't mind these discussions, thought them inevitable, really, and said that his parents were understanding, if disappointed. However, he found interest from outsiders, rather than family members, far more unwelcome and obtrusive: 'Certainly Katy gets it more than me. But a colleague at work shocked me by asking over drinks one Friday "if things were all right for us both in that department". When I said neither of us wanted children, he didn't even hesitate before telling me that I had no idea what I was missing, and that when I was a little more settled I'd change my mind. We'd both had a few pints and it got quite heated. At one point I said I took real exception to his "settled" comment, because I'd been with Katy for eight years and in that time he'd been with three women. He said he'd always thought I was immature for my age, which just made me laugh.'

David isn't alone in experiencing this. Both men and women who choose not to have children are often perceived as immature.[14] A doctoral thesis, *Mental Health Professionals' Perceptions of Voluntarily Childless Couples*, summarizes the issue thus: 'Because becoming a parent is treated as an accomplishment of adulthood, an individual who refuses to become a parent may be viewed as not wanting to "grow up". A basic principle of parenthood is that, in order to raise a child effectively, one cannot be a child. Should an individual express refusal to become a parent, a prevailing assumption about that person is that he or she lacks the capabilities required of an effective parent, including a sense of responsibility and nurturance.'[15]

Another of my own informants found the assumption of immaturity ironic, given that the reason he didn't want children was financial insecurity – he felt that his job, which he loved and did not want to change, just wasn't secure enough to bring up a child – and that by choosing not to procreate he was being more responsible than someone who went ahead and had a family, despite not being in a good position to do so.

Belief that parenthood is a rite of passage is prevalent in many countries and cultures. In the case of my Western informants, generally only those who are voluntarily childless, rather than those who have had no agency, are labelled as immature. Yet in India, in Bangladesh, in parts of Africa, the act of having a child is perceived as unlocking the gateway to adulthood for both genders. Not having a child, as we have seen, regardless of whether it is intentional or not, diminishes your role in society, infantilizes you, renders you unfit to take part as a fully mature man or woman. This may manifest itself in very practical ways – infertile women being returned to their parents' home, a man being barred from a ritual until he has a son.

Those Who Choose: The LGBT Community

For those in the lesbian, gay, bisexual and transgender community, the question of choice has a further layer of complication because of the practical difficulties involved in making a child. With a paucity of studies focusing on the experience of the child-free LGBT couple, perception of the experience tends to be anecdotal.

Eric Heinze, Professor of Law and Humanities at Queen Mary College, London, commented that, regarding children, he had never felt the 'quasi existential need for them that some people feel, both men and women, gay and straight'. Heinze acknowledged that, while people are generally less likely to comment on a gay man's childless state, there is still a perception that someone without offspring just cannot understand basic life situations: '"You can't really understand

X until you've had kids", which to me sounds like a cabby saying, "You can't really understand London unless you drive a cab."[16] However, he suspects that some gay men, even if the situation is rarer nowadays, didn't commit to a gay identity because 'their need for children within a conventional household is even stronger than their need for sex or erotic partnership, and they would therefore rather pass as straight to ensure a standard type of family life.'

Antony, who lives in South London, told the tragic story of his brother's suicide, which bore this out: 'I sometimes wonder, if I were younger, if I might want children. My brother, who was also gay but closeted, always wanted children, and this was perhaps a small part of his many great sadnesses that led to his death from suicide at thirty-four. Though I would hesitate to make a strong link there. It was very complicated. But he was certainly desirous of a heteronormative life . . . (which for him included a family).'[17]

Like Heinze, Antony hadn't felt a longing for children himself, but he did express regret that he had missed out on 'a grounding that people find through having children – or strong faith – that links them to society'. This sense of a link between parenting, faith and society seems to mirror traditional viewpoints, in the sense that a woman who is childless may not be allowed to take part in many community activities. But there is also a practical aspect. People with children congregate in nurseries and schools and share the same concerns, which also affect society as a whole. We all benefit from having a new generation who is well educated and socially aware; we all benefit from having a young work force, from having creative, constructive, engaged people around us. Parents share teacher reports, as my parents did, school performance tables, hopes, fears and dreams for someone they have brought into the world. Parenting is integral to society; it is understandable that anyone without a child may feel left out. And these gatherings are similar to religious ones, where people come together, united by a common purpose and belief, in a church, a synagogue, a temple.

The practical difficulties of having children as a gay man, the necessity for arrangements with third parties, are also a significant factor. Antony reflected: 'I also see friends who have gone to great lengths to have children with female friends and I have seen how complex their relationships have become – all sorts of gender issues, and strongly expressed rights of the mother, for example.'

Rena and Billy, a lesbian couple from Virginia, decided against having children in part because of the need to have a third party involved as a donor, but also because they had ambitions to travel widely and felt that children wouldn't fit in with their intended lifestyle. Their choice met with active approval, although not for reasons that reassured them. Rena elaborated: 'My aunt actually said, "Just as well – a child needs a father", and someone we had thought of as a friend said it would be selfish to bring a child up in such an "abnormal" – she actually used that word – family environment.'

There was almost unanimous agreement, though, from all of my interviewees that a childless gay couple was unlikely to meet the same level of comment and questioning as a heterosexual one. The heteronormative lifestyle carries an expectation of children that is absent outside of it.

Child-free: Voluntary Sterilization

In the UK sterilization as a method of contraception has been declining in popularity, from 40,000 instances in the 1970s to just 8,000 in 2015, probably in part due to the fact that the procedure is now more difficult to get on the NHS and waiting lists can be long. But in the US male and female sterilization is still the most commonly used method across the country.[18] It was, and still is, regarded by the medical establishments as best employed by people who already have a family or who are over thirty years of age. But among those who choose the child-free life, a growing number of young people in the West are seeking sterilization. Often these men and women do not wish to have to take contraceptive precautions, or do not believe in their efficacy to prevent parenthood. Their reasons for not having children do not differ from those of other child-free men and women – they include lifestyle preference, independence, and concerns over their own mental stability – yet often they report a lack of understanding and support from their healthcare provider.

The procedures themselves – tubal ligation for a woman, and vasectomy for a man –carry minimal risk, but offer freedom from what this group see as the threat of pregnancy, whether it is making someone pregnant or being with child. However, among women who seek sterilization, there is a perceived difference in the availability of the procedure for young men who wish to be sterilized and for women. In the UK the Marie Stopes clinics report a huge rise in the number of young women seeking the procedure privately, presumably because they cannot get it on the NHS.

Journalist Holly Brockwell has written widely about her own four-year battle to have the operation performed by the NHS and suffered a good deal of criticism as a result, with online commenters going as far as to say she shouldn't have sex if she doesn't want to reproduce. Brockwell believes her experience illustrates a strong gender bias, with men much more likely to convince medical practitioners of their decision to be sterilized at an earlier age.[19]

In the US, while sterilization has been legal for women over twenty-one since 1974, applying to have it done can be difficult, with few doctors prepared to carry out the procedure on childless women in their twenties.[20] The American College of Obstetricians and Gynaecologists (ACOG) carried out a comprehensive review in 2008 and have regularly issued policy statements since.[21] The 2014 statement includes the recommendation that 'women who have completed their childbearing are candidates for sterilization' but there is no ruling for women who have not yet begun their childbearing. Ethical questions focus on the issue of regret. ACOG research shows that 26 per cent of women will regret a sterilization, as opposed to fewer than 5 per cent of men, and that the number of young women under thirty who end up regretting their decision is double that of older women.[22] Sterilization also has a chequered history in North America, and it may be that the forcible sterilizations of the last century haunt the collective memory of those who would be performing the surgery. However, those demanding sterilization because it is their preferred contraceptive method argue it should be their 'right to choose', and question why any doctor should deny something when they know it is what they want.[23]

The medical ethics of sterilizing 'young, competent and

childless adults' is the subject of an academic paper by two British experts, Piers Benn, a lecturer in medical ethics and law, and Martin Lupton, a consultant in obstetrics and gynaecology.[24] They present the case of a twenty-six-year-old woman, the manager of a legal practice in London, who applied for surgical sterilization. Her reasons included a heart defect and a fear of related complications during pregnancy, but the gynaecologist assured her that the risks could be mitigated. Her other reasons remained, though – her desire to travel, the risk to her financial position, her lack of desire to become a mother. However, for me what was most interesting was her rejection of the doctor's suggestion that she ask her partner of five years to have a vasectomy instead. She said that he was only twenty-five, and if she died prematurely he might meet another woman who did want to have children. Yet she did not seem to consider the other possibility, that her partner might die or separate from her, and that she herself might meet and become involved with someone who wanted children.

The gynaecologist remained doubtful that sterilization was the best option, citing the regret commonly experienced by younger women and those who changed their relationship, so he sought a second opinion. The Hippocratic tradition bears the responsibility of 'above all, do no harm', and arguably reducing the natural functions of one's body in any way might be seen as doing harm. The conflict then arises between the oath and what the patient regards as a procedure that will enhance their life. Benn and Lupton look at this dilemma by weighing up the wishes and perceived needs of the patient with the doctor's assessment of the situation. Patient autonomy – the patient's right to determine their own course treatment and make their own decisions about their own body – is a growing feature of medicine, but a gynaecologist may feel that, based on his or her knowledge and understanding of the circumstances, a patient is making the wrong long-term decision. Specifically, the patient's present interests may not be in their best interests. How, then, can a doctor be expected to act against something he or she perceives as detrimental to the future of the patient? Is there more to making a decision that overrides the patient's current wishes than just paternalism?

Bri Seeley, an author and life coach, has written about how she first asked to be sterilized at the age of twenty-four and was continually refused until shortly before her thirtieth birthday, when she sidestepped her own physician and researched her position online. For Seeley, the decision to be childless had been a constant throughout her life. She had not named unborn babies with her friends at school and college; she had never had any inclination to have children. During her teens and twenties, her focus and ambitions did not include motherhood, so when people repeatedly asked, 'What if you change your mind?' she felt that she was being judged for not wanting to do something that society expected of her. Particularly galling for her, as for Holly Brockwell, was the gender difference – the examples of men as young as twenty-one who had managed to secure vasectomies. 'What is the difference,' she writes, 'from an adult man deciding he doesn't want to procreate and an adult woman making the same choice? Why can't I be the one to decide what's best for my life?'[25]

Five years have passed since Seeley was finally sterilized. She has not stopped questioning the obstacles that she had to

face, nor the attitude of people around her who continue to
question her decision. For her the choice was an obvious one:

    'I had been on contraception since the age of eighteen.
And by the time I turned twenty-nine, the hormones in the
birth control were no longer working for my body. I could
not imagine another thirty years taking this pill – a pill that
was messing with my body chemistry and wasn't even 100
per cent effective. I knew that I did not want children and
continuing to make temporary fixes to my situation – a
situation where I desired permanence – just did not make
sense. And while it may appear that birth control is the
easier method, I actually found my particular procedure to
be easier. It lasted all of five minutes, required five hours of
recovery, and is permanent.'

When asked how she would feel if she entered into a
relationship with someone who was desperate to have children, she is adamant that this question only serves to highlight what she sees as a much bigger issue: 'that of women
compromising their values to reach the "holy grail" of falling
in love'. For Seeley, a 'truly aligned' life partner would never
expect her to be someone she wasn't.

Such choices outside of reproductive norms attract vitriol.
In response to a *Huffington Post* article about Seeley's decision,
one man commented 'You are going to die alone.' But being
in touch with what she really wants from life has given her
strength in the face of such pronouncements: 'My role in life
is not specifically to take a stand for fertility. My role in life
is that of empowering people in themselves, their choices,
and their desires. Sharing this story of mine is one of many
examples of how I have chosen to take a stand for myself,
my desires, and my right to live out the life I wish.'

Seeley's arguments are convincing and engaging. However, is the discrepancy she perceives between society's willingness to allow a man to control his fertility and to allow her to do so the same in the UK? In 2017 the NHS Choices website stated for both male and female sterilization that 'Surgeons are more willing to perform sterilization when men/women are over thirty years old.'[26] Certainly, just two years earlier, in 2015, an Oxford University blog on Practical Ethics noted that the same NHS website mentioned the age limit only with regard to female patients, so the site may have been updated to reflect a gender equity that was less evident in practice.[27]

Is it that a man is thought to be surer in his mind at a younger age? Or is his sexuality seen as something he might need help to control? In some cultures women are expected to cover up completely to protect them from men's desire, from lust that is characterized as a wild, primeval thing; a man's inability to control himself in the face of a scantily clad woman is not a sign of weakness but of his burgeoning manhood. In the West this attitude manifests itself in newspaper reports and, until very recently, in legal cases where a woman is deemed to have deserved whatever assault she suffered because of her clothing or behaviour – she enticed him, led him on, when in fact her role was to help him to keep his lust in check. In 2011, following a series of sexual assaults in Brooklyn, women were advised by the police not to wear shorts or 'too short' skirts.[28]

In her article 'Provocative Dress and Sexual Responsibility' Jessica Wolfendale, from the University of West Virginia, cites polls that highlight the view that women, rather than men, must take responsibility for men's sexuality. For example, a study in Brazil found that 58.5 per cent of those surveyed agreed with the statement: 'Women who wear tight-fitting clothes deserve it when they are attacked.'[29]

The state's willingness to help a man seeking sterilization mirrors this attitude: it must help men to control the possible outcome of their desire, in this instance unwanted children, whereas with women, fertility itself, and the prospect of an unwanted child, help to keep their sexuality in check. Sterilization allows women to participate freely in sexual relations without the worry of contraception and for some, including several faith groups, that is an undesirable outcome.

Jonny Pugh, a research fellow in practical ethics at Oxford University, suggests that this 'paternalistic desire to ensure women prioritise fertility over what they may regard as wanton hedonism' is the less benevolent interpretation of the medical establishment's reluctance to sterilize young women.[30] The kinder interpretation assumes that a doctor is concerned with a woman being settled and sure of her decision at such a young age. However, if the same issues do not apply absolutely equally to a man of the same age who is seeking sterilization, it implies that women are regarded as less reliable in their choices and more likely to change their mind about the option of having children.

Of all the groups I considered, this was the one I found it most difficult to relate to. The women's motivations for seeking sterilization were almost always compelling, intelligent and considered, and it upset me greatly to see the extent of gender inequality, but asking a health professional to irrevocably prevent your body functioning in the way it was designed to do, rather than to cure or heal something that was amiss, troubled me. In 2014, Seeley wrote in the

Huffington Post: 'The decision to not have children does not make us less than women who choose to be mothers. Yes, we are all born with the biology to give birth, but we're not all meant to be mothers.'[31] I realized that what was missing for me was perspective. There was an assumption that fertility was something that everyone had, but that some people might not want; they should therefore be able to choose to lose it permanently, and we as a society should pay for that decision.

As an infertile person, I only feel relief if I hear that someone is voluntarily childless, that they had normative bodily function and chose not to reproduce rather than being the victim to a disobedient body. Yet the presumption of fertility was made too easily and quickly, the workings of a healthy body discussed as a problem, a kind of anti-health, rather than restoration or mending. But if this was the reluctant surgeon's dilemma, as it was my tentative doubt, it should apply equally to men and women.

Child-free: GINKS

The hashtag #Gink is all-pervasive on websites that discuss the child-free. In North America 'gink' can mean 'a foolish person', and initially I wondered if I had missed a recent web war of words between the child-free and the childless – those skirmishes that crop up from time to time and fizzle out as the comments degenerate into ad hominem attacks and playground insults. But it is an acronym that stands for 'Green Inclinations, No Kids'. The term was first used by Lisa Hymas, senior editor at *Grist*, who has a blog solely devoted to Gink Think, where she defies 'the pro-natal bias that runs deep'.

We are all encouraged to recycle rubbish, cycle to work, mind our carbon footprint, but, as Hymas points out, the most effective way (even when all the possibles are aggregated) to avoid contributing to the destruction of our environment is not to have a child. Hymas doesn't proselytize that others should stop having children to support her green campaigning, but she does encourage debate and feels that her own choice is not a sacrifice but, rather, an indulgence that allows her to do what is best for the planet. Hymas explains: 'I've spent my life on environmental issues, so for me it was just about connecting the dots. But everyone should be able to make their own decisions about their reproduction. Everyone should have easy access to the tools to enable them to do so.'[32]

Anna Williams, a London-based counsellor, has similar beliefs. 'My feeling is that basically people are condemning their child to an environmental disaster.' When I probe further, she is explicit: 'People need to have smaller families. But also to really think about why they want a child and to understand what kind of a world they are bringing that child into. Having children is the biggest carbon footprint you can make.' She adds that population growth isn't stabilizing and that we are 'adding 240,000 people each day'.[33]

The environmental impact of having children is exacerbated by Western lifestyles. An Oregon State University study showed that in the United States, 'the carbon legacy and greenhouse gas impact of an extra child is almost twenty times more important than some of the other environmentally sensitive practices people might employ their entire lives –

things like driving a high-mileage car, recycling, or using energy-efficient appliances and light bulbs.'[34]

Hymas concurs: 'As a financially comfortable American, I use a lot of stuff and take up a lot of room. My carbon footprint is more than 200 times bigger than an average Ethiopian's, and more than twelve times bigger than an average Indian's, and twice as big as an average Brit's.[35]

Williams's and Hymas's position seems a direct challenge to the one which is more prevalent in the media: child-free people are selfish. I've heard it often enough in my own life, generally formed as a question, as if that will some-how lessen the offensiveness of the notion. But even Pope Francis, as mentioned above, has openly expressed this opinion, so its popularity and prevalence aren't surprising at all: 'A society with a greedy generation, that doesn't want to surround itself with children, that considers them above all worrisome, a weight, a risk, is a depressed society.'[36] For the GINKS, too much human life is using up our limited supplies of energy. The resources of the planet are finite. Society may well be enriched, but what of the earth that sustains it?

Mary Evans is a British academic with three children.[37] She is environmentally active, supports the Green Party, cycles to work in London and does not own a car. What does she think of this reasoning? Did she ever think that her green activism might be at odds with her decision to have three children? 'No, not at all – perhaps, just perhaps, by raising children who are similarly aware I can help preserve the planet for longer.' Yet this hope rests on the assumption that her children will share her values and concerns. There are no guarantees that the child of a green activist won't become someone who loathes trains, refuses to recycle and drives the car short distances to avoid walking.

Motivation is an intriguing thing. I am further irritated when a green-aware colleague suggests that the answer to population control is simply a matter of providing contraception to developing countries. Of course, it's not a new idea, but I am annoyed that the onus to save the planet has apparently fallen on those doing least damage to it. Providing contraceptives to a society where a lack of progeny will result in starvation and poverty in your later years, or where the number of children you have dictates your value in a community, is not a solution to the fundamental issue of overconsumption.

Population Matters, a London-based organization, campaigns to encourage smaller families. It too focuses on the environmental benefits of having small families. Its philosophy is neo-Malthusian, heeding the warning of Thomas Malthus in 1798 that the population will just keep growing until it is halted 'by misery and vice'.[38] But while it shows an appreciation that empowering women and girls in developing countries is an essential part of change as much as access to free contraception, it keeps the weight of responsibility firmly with those who can already choose. The Population Matters website states, 'Where we already have the choice to determine the size of our families, we must exercise that choice freely and mindfully. A just and stable transition to sustainable numbers can only occur gradually and through choice.'[39]

Aubrey Manning, Emeritus Professor of Natural History at the University of Edinburgh and a patron of Population Matters, is quoted as saying, 'Looking across the world at present it is obvious to anybody with even slight biological knowledge that human numbers are out of balance.' Sir David Attenborough is also a patron and in his lecture to the RSA (Royal Society for the Encouragement of Arts, Manufactures and Commerce) in 2011, he spoke openly about the dangers of overpopulation. 'The unprecedented increase of the number of human beings on the planet' is not sustainable. Attenborough urged that the issue of population control should take its place alongside climate change and that what he sees as the current taboo around discussing population control should be dropped; educated people need to 'break the taboo in private and in public' so that 'wherever and whenever you speak of environment [you] bring up the issue of population control'.

Population Matters has a remit that goes beyond the promotion of smaller families. The organization is also active in women's issues such as FGM as well as child and forced marriages, arguing that women who have more control over their lives will also be able to choose when and if to have children. However, its specified goals include asking governments to integrate 'population projections into their planning and policies, and to promote smaller families'.

This is, of course, the opposite of the sinister pronatalist policies of Iran and North Korea, but is redolent of the Chinese solution, where smaller families were promoted and then enforced, which, as we saw in an earlier chapter, has had negative consequences too. The idea of state population control sits uneasily on the brink of allowing government organizations to influence choices that belong in the domain of free will. So what other factors might be used to encourage and promote smaller families?

In his lecture, Attenborough specifically warned against the dangers of enforced population control, emphasizing that people must retain the right to have as many children as they want, but that a programme of education and awareness of 'how much trouble larger families can cause', coupled with free and easy access to contraception, could help steer them towards the right choice – the only one that was environmentally feasible.

Hymas shares this view: 'We do need large-scale, societal solutions. Most people, given the tools and means to control their fertility, don't have very large families. I don't think governments should be telling people how many children to have. They need the tools to make the choice.'[40] When I asked her what some of the solutions might be, Hymas cited attempts to use soap-opera plots to influence family planning in areas where population growth, overcrowding and poverty were rising rapidly. Research from the University of Oxford catalogues the success of these experiments right from their earliest days. The first *telenovela* with a plot designed to encourage smaller families was shown in Mexico in the late 1970s.[41]

Once upon a time Amanda, Raquel and Esperanza were three happy-going young women growing up in Tacubaya in Mexico City. However, the three sisters' lives have become very different since marrying and having their own families. Amanda is a middle-class professional. She's had three children, all planned, and has raised them in a harmonious atmosphere. However, her happy family will soon be shattered when she learns her husband has terminal cancer. Raquel is a spoiled rich woman, who only has one son. She's refused to give her husband more children for fear that they will destroy her body. Her only child grows unloved and neglected. Esperanza married a promising young man, but she did not believe in contraceptives, so her family grew too large for comfort. Because her husband's salary is not enough to support them, Esperanza and her children, several of whom are psychotic and potential criminals, must move into a rundown shack, where they cohabit in squalor and constant bickering.

In 1977 the telenovela *Acompáñame* was a huge success, with calls to the National Planning Office in Mexico increasing from none at all to an average of 500 calls each month. Following one plot line, 2,000 women registered as volunteers in the National Program of Family Planning, and more than 560,000 women enrolled in local family-planning clinics, 33 per cent up on the previous year.[42] A series of further soaps to convey a family-planning message were commissioned and shown in the following decades. Thomas Donnelly from the United States Agency for International Development stated in 2009 that 'The Televisa family-planning soap operas have made the single most powerful contribution to the Mexican population success story'.[43]

Today the fertility rate in Mexico, representing the number of children a woman has in her lifetime, has dropped to an all-time low.[44]

However, similar attempts to influence family size through television dramas have been much less successful in India. *Hum Log* (*People Like Us*) was the first soap opera to promote a social message in India. Viewers sent more than 400,000 letters to an address given in an epilogue at the end of each show, which related the storyline to viewers' lives. These letters were addressed not only to the actors but to the characters portrayed. Research into 500 of the letters showed a very positive reaction – '92 per cent were influenced in a pro-social direction' – but only 7 per cent changed their behaviour as a result.[45] This was partly because of a lack of inter-institutional cooperation between the media, public health groups and voluntary organizations, but also because the underlying social issues to do with the position of women in the family, women's emancipation and the high value placed on fertility, were not addressed properly.

In a recent piece for *Foreign Policy* magazine, the academics Travis Rieder and Rebecca Kukla discuss the ethics of having children given the environmental implications of doing so. Rieder suggests that 'preference-adjusting campaigns', such as the Mexican *telenovelas*, may be an alternative to draconian state control. Kukla stresses that this might not counter the 'unquestioned assumption that it's a woman's job to manage reproduction'; there is a need to empower men to have more informed and proactive involvement.[46]

Clearly, any attempts to limit family size will first have to address social and cultural issues that foster large families, as well as providing easy access to contraceptive methods.

Childless for God

Historically, Christianity has always offered alternative paths for women. During medieval times, the Beguines in northern Europe did not live under the guardianship of a man, as their contemporaries did, nor were they bound by the formal vows of a nun. Christian mystics such as Joan of Arc and Hildegard of Bingen were driven by their faith to challenge gender-based bias of their capabilities and role.

Because childbearing is seen by many as the pinnacle of a woman's achievement, and many churches endorse this view, the choice to live a celibate life because of faith intrigues me. I am curious to know about the conflict between, for example, the honouring of motherhood in the contemporary practice of many Christian faiths, and the abnegation of it in favour of God.

A Salesian nun from New Jersey in the United States, Sister Brittany, shares her own views and experience with me. She is very explicit about how she sees herself: 'I'm not childless. As a nun, I'm a spiritual mother to many.' She follows up by sending me links to articles and items about 'spiritual motherhood', a topic that the church is seeing more and more frequently in retreats and forums and faith groups. A Carmelite website displays the following definition: 'Spiritual motherhood is about caring and self-giving. It is other-focused. Recessed in the nooks and crannies of our daily lives, if we open our eyes, we discover people who need spiritual nurturing, affirmation, and guidance, and don't receive it. This is spiritual motherhood, and it isn't only for biological mothers . . . Spiritual motherhood is about nurturing life.[47]

Rather than choosing not to have children as a result of religious faith, the idea is that you are opting to have more children, albeit spiritual ones, whom you can lead and guide and cherish. 'The world sees what the religious woman gives up . . . marriage to one man, a family of her own children. The religious woman sees what she receives, Christ as her spouse, and all the peoples of the world as her children. Marriage to Christ did not free her *from* a family but *for* His family.'[48]

In 2013 Pope Francis spoke of 'fertile chastity' and the duty of those in the religious life to bring spiritual children to the church. Nuns were to be 'mothers not spinsters'. Thus the language used by the church manages to align two very contradictory positions: that motherhood is the highest calling for a woman, and yet those who devote themselves to the world are spiritually childless.

When Sister Brittany shared her experience with me, it was immediately obvious that she rejoiced in her vocation and the work that she carried out as a result of it, but I wondered if there was ever a fleeting moment when not giving birth to a child was something she regretted or wished for. She replied, 'Do I feel I am a mother? Yes. I have never given birth, nor shall I ever, as far as I know. Of course, there is a certain painful sense tied into that renunciation of physical "birth giving", for part of me does long to see my face mirrored in that of a child whom I have created with my husband through love – what an incredible mystery children are!'[49]

Sister Brittany spoke of the *charism* of motherhood, from the Greek *kharisima*, meaning gift or grace. She described it as an innate form of loving that might apply equally to men in relationship to fatherhood. A woman may manifest *charism* differently, depending on role, vocation, job, culture; the qualities of 'interiority, reflection, nurturing and protecting life within herself, giving of herself to sustain another', all traditionally associated with motherhood, are nevertheless there even if a woman's situation does not give her the opportunity to develop them. And even if she doesn't 'deepen and develop' these characteristics, it is through them that she relates to others. Sister Brittany was unequivocal:

'Every day I relate as a mother to many people. I nurture the development of my students, guard them in their sorrows and console them. I sacrifice my body for their good in my labours and tears for them. I carry each of them in "the womb of my heart", offering them the sustenance of my prayers and loving thoughts, that they might be sustained in physical and spiritual life. I could go on, but I think you are starting to understand my point. I am a mother. A spiritual mother, but a mother nonetheless.[50]

For Sister Brittany, the Catholic tradition does not limit mothering to the experience of birth. After all: 'To say that a woman is only a mother if she gives physical birth is very limiting of womanhood; it's like a part of her remains undeveloped and dormant . . . how sad! What of those women who are unable to conceive but care for others – are they not motherly? What of those women who have lost their children – do they cease to be mothers? What of those women who embrace a vocation (lifestyle) like mine – are we somehow stunted in our womanhood?'[51]

I found other cases within the Catholic church where motherhood in this metaphorical sense extended beyond the relationship between a nun and her flock. Indeed, a woman who does not have a religious vocation can also choose to be a spiritual mother to a priest. In 2007 the Vatican issued a document entitled *Eucharistic Adoration for the Sanctification of Priests and Spiritual Motherhood*: 'The vocation to be a spiritual mother for priests is largely unknown, scarcely understood and, consequently, rarely lived, notwithstanding its fundamental importance.'[52] This role is open to all devout, practising women, whether 'single, married or in the consecrated life'. The Apostolate of the Spiritual Mothers of Priests in Ottawa inducts women following a two-day formation process before making a life offering. The spiritual mother prays for a parish priest as well as bishops and new vocations, and during her welcoming receives a letter from her particular 'priest son'. This too offers an alternative route to motherhood within the church.

In her book *Reconceiving Women*, Mardy Ireland argues that different and conflicting theories of psychology share a commonality in their assertion that a 'woman's reproductive capacity shapes her mental life', but she does not explore the idea that a woman's capacity to give birth is not the same as her 'capacity to produce biological children'.[53] Yet motherhood, either in its physical or its spiritual sense, is a central tenet of the church, and intrinsic to the role of women in society. While Sister Brittany thought it limiting to think of women as mothers only when they have physically given birth, I wondered why we have to consider them as any kind of mother. Isn't it enough to be a woman? What is it about the role of mother that means we have to attain it, whatever the difficulties, whatever the form? This symbolic, non-physical motherhood gives the impression of being a redemptive thing, protection against the fate that is too awful to acknowledge – that of never being any kind of mother at all.

I spoke, in confidence, with Mary, a former nun from southern Italy, who later agreed I could use her remarks if I protected her identity.[54] She had left the church to marry, both because she had fallen in love and because she longed for a child. 'If I'm honest,' she said, 'the longing started out as my penance, something I offered up to God, but when I met Martin, I felt I had been called in another way.' But Mary wasn't able to have children; she made contact with me in response to a call to hear from women who were childless and did not wish to be. Her husband is separated from her and, although they are not divorced, has had a child with another woman. For Mary, it seems as if she is being punished. 'I know it's not logical, but that's how I feel. I'm neither a spiritual mother nor a real mother. I have no value. Somehow I confused God's calling with my own desire. I still have the support of the church and my local priest has been very kind, but I know I am becoming a bitter woman. When I see [Martin] with his son, I resent the child, his child. God forgive me, but I do.'

The Catholic tradition is far from alone in correlating a woman's value with her role as a mother. To cite just one example, when women were welcomed into Buddhist holy orders in India, the monasteries offered a haven for childless women who had been shunned by their village or town, as well as a refuge for those whose children had died and were no longer deemed to be of any worth to Brahmin society. But the monastic life that they followed was still apart from everyday life, from community decision-making, and thus the strictures of the holy life perpetuated the predominant belief that a childless woman no longer had a role in her community.[55]

Childless by Circumstance, and Happy About It

In the chapter 'Those Who Long' we saw that the phrase 'childless by circumstance' is used by some people who have not had children because of particular life events

that conspired against the possibility – for example, acting
as a carer for another family member and delaying having
children, but alas leaving it too late. However, some of those
who find themselves in this situation embrace their childless
state and do not regard it as something to be lamented. It
is not a majority position; most people who are child-free
make a very conscious decision to be so, as a survey by
the universities of Maine and Massachusetts showed: participants felt that their decision was well thought out and
deliberate, perhaps more so than the choice to have children
often was.[56]

The childless by circumstance are among the most vocal
on social media. Many of them are seeking to improve life
for all those who are childless, regardless of how they came
to be so. In the United States they often refer to themselves as
'childless by chance', and one of the most common reasons
is not having found the right partner – either one who wants
children or anyone at all.

The American author Melanie Notkin deplores the
prevalence of stereotypes and misconceptions about why a
woman doesn't have children. There's a general feeling 'that
they're too picky in love – or not picky enough; that they're
too careless (about their fertility) or too serious (about their
careers).'[57] A successful professional woman who is also a
mother of two is lauded for managing to achieve so much;
the woman who hasn't given birth has done less, although if
she has been especially high-achieving she may be marked
as someone who has forgone the chance of children to focus
on her career. In Carolyn Morrell's book *Unwomanly Conduct*,
Ellen, aged forty-three, insists: 'Forgo being a mother? There
have been so many other things in my life that I don't see it as

forgoing, because it was a choice that gradually evolved, and it wasn't as if I sat there and said, "I can either be a physician or a mother." I was going to be a physician. Whether I was going to be a mother down the road I wasn't sure.'[58] The irony is that a childless woman who is dismissed as too interested in her career to give birth may have developed her work focus as compensation for the fact that she is childless but does not wish to be.

Vicky Smith, from London, is happy with her child-free life now, but it isn't the one she expected she would have. A successful lawyer, now in her forties, Vicky was divorced when she was in her twenties. She freely acknowledges that she didn't want to have children as young as that, but she always assumed that in her thirties she would meet someone, settle down, and juggle career and child care in the way that so many of her contemporaries do. Her husband wasn't keen to have a family at all and Vicky explains that, while it was not the only reason for the split, it was certainly a big contributing factor. 'By the time I was thirty I started really trying to find someone. I took the same attitude that I had towards my legal studies – the idea that if you put enough effort into it, you'll get there. I did blind dates, a bit of internet dating, though it wasn't as big then as it is now, and I went out a lot. After I finished work I would always be the one saying, let's go to the pub, or, let's see a show. I thought I was never going to meet anyone sitting at home. I really envied my colleagues who were all sorted – you know, not having to desperately get out all the time on the off-chance of finding Mr Right, but instead staying in with the TV and their husbands, and a bit later their kids. It was exhausting. I couldn't do it now. Oh, I had a few relationships, but none of them worked out, and when I grew tired of the whole thing and realized I was getting a bit old to have children, I focussed on my work. I changed job when I was in my late thirties to one that I knew was more demanding. It's been a godsend. I don't have time for all the gallivanting and, in fact, though it's too late for me to have children now, I do have a lovely, caring partner, who was the friend of a colleague's client, of all things.[59]

Her story resonated with me. If I hadn't met my husband, I would have felt very differently about having children. I certainly wouldn't have had the courage to try on my own, as so many other women do. Vicky, like Notkin and almost all of the informants interviewed by Morrell, also felt that people somehow 'blamed her career' for her childlessness, and found it both irritating and ill-considered.

Children, or the lack of them, are inextricably linked to the sex act and to our own experience of it. In their book *Infertility Around the Globe*, Marcia Inhorn and Frank Van Balen point out that 'when couples remain childless, issues of sexual "failure" come to the fore'.[60] This makes it a subject that is not easily discussed. When questioned in a social situation, a childless person might choose to focus on their career choice and to move away from a discussion of their relationship history, saying, 'I chose a career over children', rather than, 'I never found the right partner', or some other personal explanation. Individuals who fear stigma will often seek to control information, especially when the child-free have their privacy invaded by people with whom they are not well acquainted questioning their status: 'To tell or not to tell, to let on or not to let on, to lie or not to lie, and in each case to whom, when and where.'[61]

Furthermore Dr Kristin Park, a sociologist at the University of Westminster, has noted how the child-free will often seek to redefine their situation to listeners in a proactive way. This may both challenge 'parenthood prescription' and also reaffirm the speaker's value and contribution to greater society. Studies and surveys would therefore need to be anonymous to present a more open and truer account, one that was free from fear of social judgement.[62]

A Short Note on Femininity
and Womanhood

The notion of womanhood, of what is feminine, perplexes me. I began bleeding when I was eleven but I was clearly still a girl. Yet in some places that would mark my passage to adulthood. In others I would only gain the role of woman with the birth of my first child. Without pregnancy, I would be stunted. My development broken off, indefinitely interrupted.

I only recently read the celebrated feminist essay 'Laugh of the Medusa' by Hélène Cixous. It was published in 1975 and, in a dismissive footnote, Cixous says the only women to have written works which might be called feminine in France in the twentieth century are Colette and Marguerite Duras.[1] They are both mothers. She excludes Simone De Beauvoir, Simone Weil and Anaïs Nin, who were not.

Cixous wrote her essay two years after Nin had already written of the relationship between a woman's body, her sensory perception of the world through it, and her writing. I have loved Nin since I was a teenager; for me it is an almost unforgiveable slight. Admittedly, the work that moves me most was published after Cixous wrote her essay. The publication of Nin's unexpurgated diary, *Incest*, was held back until most of the people who populate it were dead. The book contains a conversation she has with her unborn child in August 1934, immediately before she aborts the foetus. It is surely *feminine*, if such a thing can be defined. I prefer the word 'womanly', though. *Feminine* is too redolent, somehow, of lace and frills and giggling. Women bleed and piss and shit. They may give birth, push bloodied children from their gaping holes; they may have someone drag or suck out an unborn, unwanted body because it was not their choice for it to be inside them; their womb might never grow anything at all.

Nin's awful, gut-wrenching, harrowing description of a very late abortion contains some of the most powerful passages in literature. It is just as *womanly* as writing on the miracle of childbirth. I read: 'The child is not a child; it is a demon lying half-choked between my legs, keeping me from living, strangling me, showing only its head until I die in its grasp.' Or: 'The womb is stirring and dilating. Drum, drum, drum, drum. "I am ready!" The nurse puts her knee on my stomach. There is blood in my eyes, blood, blood. A tunnel. I push into this tunnel. I bite my lips and push.'[2]

Because of Nin's abortion and her reaction to it, her biographer, Deirdre Bair, accused her of 'monstrous egotism and selfishness, horrifying in its callous indifference'.[3] In the press frenzy that followed the publication of the biography, Nin was dismissed as someone who 'lied and fornicated the way the rest of us breathe'. She was a sexual object, a dirty girl who had too much sex with the wrong men in the wrong circumstances, a bigamist, an upper-class, pampered pet with a streak of rebelliousness. Guilty of lots of child-free sex. Sex explicitly not for procreation. A 2015 article in the *Guardian*, reflecting on the events, calls the furore 'slut-shaming' before the term was invented.[4] Her biographer had character-assassinated her subject, reduced her reputation to that of an explicitly 'minor writer', while capitalizing and passing judgement on a life that was filled with debauchery. Cixous's omission of someone who had once been the toast of French literature and who was awarded the Prix Sévigné in 1971 seemed momentarily justified. But with the internet, Nin has been reborn. Despite academic misgivings over her literary merits and doubt cast on her honesty, her iconic status was restored as women reclaimed their sexuality on blogs, social media and virtual forums.[5]

Undoubtedly mendacious, but creatively so, Nin melded her own story seamlessly with fictitious elaborations and narrative enhancements. She was a mistress of her own invention. The internet is a new world where identity is a much more fluid thing and all manner of experience, beyond that which was previously deemed socially acceptable – suitably *feminine* – may be shared, even feted. Nin, her explicit writing and the way that she created her own alter ego, an avatar for the media of her time, has become far more pertinent to the future than her detractors and those who dismissed her. She was a childless woman born in 1903, whose posthumous reputation has triumphed over slut-shaming and disregard: an icon of womanhood for a new age.

A Short Note on the Voices of History

For the Ancient Egyptians, fertility was essential. The Kahun
Gynaecological Papyrus, found at El Lahun in Egypt, dates
from 1825 BC and there's a cure for infertility in it. It suggests
that you should have the infertile woman 'sit on earth smeared
with dregs of sweet beer', then stuff her mouth with dates. If
she vomits, each act of vomiting will mean a birth; if she
does not, then she 'will never give birth'. Another section
suggests that if you place 'a bundle of onions' in the woman's
vagina overnight and can smell the onions on her breath the
next morning she is fertile.[1]

Plato provides a distinctive account of the creation of
woman and her sexual desire in *Timaeus*, one of his *Dialogues*.
He links woman's desire for sexual intercourse with her
womb's desire for child-bearing. Furthermore, he relates
that if the womb is deprived of its desire, it will roam around
the woman's body like an animal and block the passages of
respiration. Barren wombs were therefore particularly given
to wandering, which seemed appropriate to me, because, for
me, the pain of endometriosis was rarely in a single fixed
place but roamed around different reproductive organs in
an unpredictable way. One day my left ovary, another my
right, sometimes my womb itself would throb as if it was
impatient to escape.

In Ancient Rome there were tangible rewards, in the

shape of wealth and promotion, for those who could father children. Pliny the Younger was adopted by his uncle, who was unable to have children, and, despite having three wives, the younger Pliny too failed to become a parent. Writing to his third wife's grandfather, Calpurnius Fabatus, he seems to blame his wife for their misfortune when Calpurnia has a miscarriage: 'Being young and inexperienced, she did not realize she was pregnant, failed to take the proper precautions, and did several things that were better left undone.' Pliny sympathizes with his elderly relative's grief at not having a 'descendant already on the way' but also asks that he thank the Gods for sparing the life of his granddaughter, who has been in grave danger as a result of the miscarriage. He is pleased that she has proved to be fertile, and consoles both himself and Calpurnius with the fact that, when they do have children, achieving office for them will be easy, given the family connections, and they will be left well provided for, with 'a well-known name and an established ancestry'.

Pliny's worries, about continuity and his ability to provide for the family he hopes for, are ageless and poignant. But children did not come and Pliny's only consolation was when the Emperor Trajan recognized his other abilities and awarded him the privileges normally granted to those who have fathered three children. He continued to love Calpurnia. Three letters remain of those he wrote to her, of which the last is most passionate: 'You would scarcely credit how much I miss you and long to see you again. My love for you is the primary cause of this longing, and the fact that we have not been used to be away from each other is the second. Hence it is that I spend a great part of my nights awake and thinking of you, and regularly at the hours when I used to visit you I find my feet carrying me – in the literal sense of the term – towards your room, and then, sick and sad at heart, and feeling as though I had been refused admittance, I turn to quit the empty threshold.'[2]

But of the women's feelings we can only speculate. The assumption is that they too longed for the children that did not come, but it is also possible that they were relieved to avoid the risk of death that so often accompanied pregnancy and birth. None of Calpurnia's letters remain; there are no hieroglyphs to tell us what became of the women who were tested with sweet beer and dates. They left no ancestors; they left no trace of their voices.

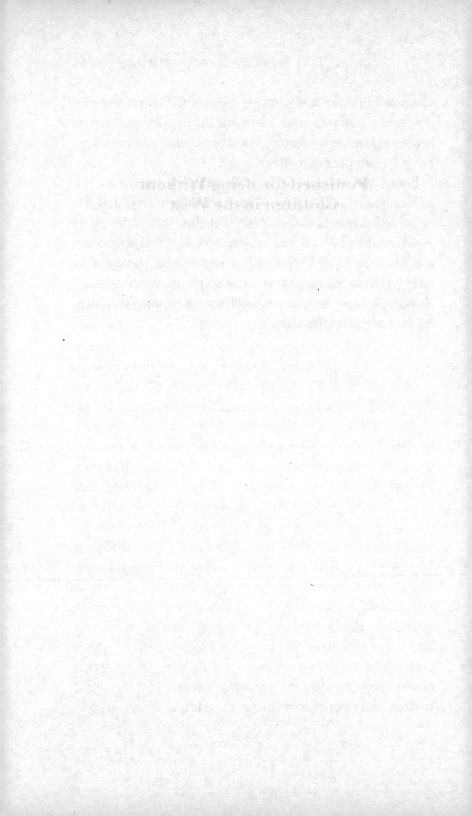

7

Punished for Being Without Children in the West

B eyond the emotional regret and deep sadness of those who wished to have children but could not, there are other societal, public issues which affect all childless and child-free people in Western culture. As well as practical matters – everything from taxation and discrimination in the workplace to old-age care and loneliness – not having children is still seen as a deviation from cultural norms, and that brings its own problems. Western society is predominantly pronatalist and the childless and child-free are often interrogated as to the reason for their state. If it then becomes known that someone is voluntarily childless, they suffer from negative stereotyping and may be regarded as 'less nurturing, socially undesirable, selfish, individualistic, irresponsible, materialistic and less mature'.[1] One qualitative academic study from the United States reported that women who choose to be child-free are usually regarded as deviant, and treated with disbelief and disregard.[2] In order to avoid this disdain, women may actively pretend to have an interest in 'one day' conceiving. Academic Gilla Shapiro's overview of the literature on the perception and reception of the child-free cites the example of a thirty-one-year-old woman who does exactly this, even with her friends, despite acknowledging their liberal values.[3] Simone de Beauvoir's arguments against seeing women as wombs in *The Second Sex* (1949) have not been accepted in the way we might expect in twenty-first-century Britain or America. There has been surprisingly little change in attitudes towards the childless by choice over the past thirty years since the first research into Western outlooks was conducted. Dr Annalucia Bays, a psychologist from Virginia Commonwealth University, argues that not only is there 'a persistence of negative perceptions of women without children in a contemporary sample of emerging US adults' but that these 'negative perceptions and emotions may result in harm from others'.[4]

Regarding women as defined by their reproductive capacity reduces both the childless and the child-free to the status of 'other'. That 'other' can then be singled out for judgement. The effect is highly marked in some societies, where it can result in exclusion and violence, but, in others, is more insidious. The more patriarchal the society, the greater the link between a woman's identity and her reproductive ability and choices.

Punished for Being Childless: Taxation

Financial disadvantages to being childless in the UK are much less often highlighted than the cost of raising a family, but they are prevalent. Recent changes to inheritance tax saw a flurry of petitions and an open letter from a law firm challenging the government for discriminating against the childless. The original law stated that if an estate was worth more than £325,000, it was subject to inheritance tax

(IHT), thus 40 per cent of the value above that threshold went to Her Majesty's Revenue and Customs. Couples could combine this allowance and pass on assets of up to £625,000 before any tax was due. From 2017, an incrementally increasing tax-exempt amount was added to this over each twelve-month period beginning at £100,000 per person, but crucially this increment was only available to those who have direct descendants to whom they will leave their inheritance.

The government was not subtle about its objective: 'This measure will reduce the burden of IHT for most families by making it easier to pass on the family home to direct descendants without a tax charge.'[5] The CEO of the law firm Latimer Hinks called the government to account in an open letter: 'It's nothing short of discrimination to say if you are childless, you will not get the same financial advantages as those who do have children, even though you have contributed to society as a tax payer by helping to pay for education, maternity leave and childcare costs.'[6] But childless and child-free discrimination tends not to be as well publicized as that which affect parents and does not garner support from those with families, no matter how blatant. A petition to end this restricted benefit gained only 607 signatures of the 100,000 needed to take the issue to parliament.[7]

In the United States the Earned Income Tax Credit (EITC) is a refundable tax credit for low-income families. It has enabled more mothers to participate in the labour force, but has either zero or negative impact for second earners in married couples or for the childless. In 2016 a low-income family with three or more children could get up to $6,269. For adults with no children, any benefit was capped at $506.

For this credit to be effective as an anti-poverty tool, it would have to address the big disparity in its applicability to those who do and do not have children. Harry Holzer, a renowned economist from Georgetown University, points out that: 'Federal and state EITC payments to low-income parents with children have expanded dramatically in recent decades, with clear benefits to the poor in terms of higher income and work effort. But few jurisdictions extend much of these benefits to low-income childless adults and non-custodial parents, who are often less-educated men. Indeed, this group has suffered greater losses in wages and has responded with greater declines in labour force activity than any other major demographic group.'[8]

The net result is that low-income, childless families without access to the EITC, or for whom it is a tiny sum, do not have enough compensation to make up for their income tax and their employee share of payroll taxes; they are effectively 'taxed into poverty'.[9]

Punished for Being Childless: Work Discrimination

While workplace discrimination against parents is an acknowledged issue with specific rights to protect mothers and fathers enshrined in law, many non-parents also experience discrimination at work. They may, for example, have to take holidays at particular times to fit in with the needs of colleagues who are mothers and fathers, or be expected to take on extra duties at evenings or weekends because childcare is not an issue for them. Laura Carroll, writing in *Fortune* magazine, sees it as a difference in perception between the 'important' work of parenting and the less-valued free time of those without children. It is part of the common assumption, also mentioned by Melanie Notkin, that 'non-parent employees can and will pick up the slack for their parent colleagues when asked'.[10] There's very little that protects their time to care for themselves and their families and enjoy work-life balance.[11]

This is seen as due to a 'cultural lag', with employers not yet understanding that the child-free and childless deserve the same right to a work-life balance as parents. Carroll also picks up on the erroneous assumption that those women without children 'must be putting their careers ahead of having kids'. Within the workplace this can lead to them being viewed as 'career-obsessed' and 'driven to climb the career ladder', when this is so rarely the case.[12] They may then be expected to take on more work or extra responsibility whether they wish it or not.

In an interview with the *New York Post*, magazine editor and writer Meghann Foye declared that having children was the 'only path that offered a modicum of flexibility'; she argued that those without children should be offered 'meternity leave', which she saw as 'a sabbatical-like break that allows women and, to a lesser degree, men to shift their focus to the part of their lives that doesn't revolve around their jobs'.[13] Foye met with an avalanche of online abuse, so much so that she was forced to cancel an appearance on *Good Morning America*. In her absence, the show's anchor and the guest speaker presenting the opposing viewpoint, Dr Janet Taylor, a psychiatrist and mother-of-four, united in their criticism. Taylor dismissed Foye's depiction of maternity leave: 'There's no question you need "me-time". But maternity leave is not a time of play, passion, or reflection. It's a time of you bonding, being sleep-deprived . . . it's all about your child. Once again, it pits moms versus non-moms. As women, we don't need that. I think it really minimizes the notion of stress and guilt for working moms. And it undermines the fact that being a mother is a twenty-four-hour, seven-day-a-week, full-time commitment, and we can't belittle that.'

Yet in her argument Taylor too was setting the childless and mothers against each other, and very specifically raising the importance of the mother's role and a woman's decision to be a mother, above the decision not to. It ignored the fundamental point of Foye's argument, one later picked up by Hannah Betts in the *Telegraph*, that having children was a lifestyle choice – hard work, no doubt, but work that you opted for – with no less or more validity than a different decision, say to travel, or to write a book.[14]

It seemed almost unbelievable that, even today, the suggestion that women who are not mothers should be entitled to a life-enhancing break met with so much derision and scorn, rather than any kind of debate, predominantly from other women, that Foye felt she had to go to ground.

For men, work discrimination may take a very particular form. In the UK the Trades Union Congress (TUC) recently investigated the position of childless men with regard to salary. They found that, on average, fathers earn a fifth more than men without children. While fathers did tend to work slightly longer hours than their child-free colleagues, the difference did not account for the large discrepancy. Citing European studies that suggest a child-free man's CV is looked on much less favourably, the general secretary of the TUC remarked, 'It says much about current attitudes that men with children are seen as more committed by employers.'[15]

Political Inclusion

In Britain election campaigns and political policy always centre around family, in particular 'hard-working families', that beloved phrase used by all political persuasions. Campaign posters will often use the words, 'As a mother I understand . . .' or, 'As a parent I can relate to . . .', the implication being that if you are not a parent, you will not be able to. It's an issue that's not limited to a particular political orientation. In 2016 Labour leadership candidate Owen Smith proclaimed, 'I'm normal – I've got a wife and three children', as part of his speech when standing against Angela Eagle, a childless lesbian. In 2016 an article in *The Times*, which mainly focused on Nicola Sturgeon's miscarriage in 2011, included a sidebar of 'childless women politicians' from a wide political spectrum.[16] It appeared one year after a *New Statesman* cover showed Dr Merkel, Nicola Sturgeon, Theresa May and Liz Kendall and asked the question, 'Why are so many successful women childless?' Sturgeon tweeted the image with the line: 'Jeezo . . . we appear to have woken up in 1965 this morning.'

In 2017 the Gatestone Institute, a prominent international think tank, published an opinion piece by the Italian journalist and author Giulio Meotti under the headline 'Europe's Childless Leaders Sleepwalking Us to Disaster'. Meotti argues that 'being a mother or a father . . . means that you have a very real stake in the future of the country you lead'. He quotes the German philosopher Rüdiger Safranski: 'for the childless, thinking in terms of the generations to come loses relevance'. It's a damning dismissal of a large number of politicians and wilfully ignores their qualifications or experience, focusing instead on their children or lack of them. It also makes the ridiculous assumption, albeit one that is far too often made, that only people with biological or adopted offspring care about what happens after their life has ended.[17]

In 2016 the Turkish president Recep Tayyip Erdoğan announced that child-free women are 'giving up on humanity'. In a speech to the Turkish Women's and Democracy Association (KADEM) Erdogan urged women to have at least three children, saying: 'A women who rejects motherhood, who refrains from being around the house, however successful her working life is, is deficient, is incomplete.'[18]

But there are signs that there may be a new understanding for those without children elsewhere. Controversially, in Australia, the Liberal Democrat Party have made the issue of inequity for the childless and child-free in society central to their politics. In a speech that began, 'Won't someone think about the childless? Politicians seem to be obsessed with families,' Senator Leyonhjelm argued that 'people without children should not be forced to subsidize people with children', and that there was 'no moral case to make them subsidize other people's choices'. He spoke for both the child-free and childless, but in the case of the latter, who had wanted children, he described the way they had to support parents financially as being 'charity in reverse'.

Raising familiar arguments that people who have received benefits when they were young are simply paying back to the next generation, he pointed out that many of them may not have received any benefits at all. Furthermore the idea that everyone should pay to raise children because they may one day require services from them (or benefit from their contribution) was ridiculed as being akin to having to pay to train a baker because one day you will want to eat bread.

When the speech was posted on YouTube, a plethora of comments highlighted the hugely disparate reaction to these proposals. One particularly poignant post, picking up on Leyonhjelm's comment about 'reverse charity', said: 'There are so many childless couples who want but cannot have children. Who have spent thousands of dollars trying to conceive with no luck and who do not meet the criteria to adopt. Parents who have had miscarriage after miscarriage. No one pays for their expenses. They have no one to lean on or fall back on and are not asking anyone for a handout. Yet, even with all of these expenses and heartaches, they are still being asked to support other people's children – this is a painful slap in the face that one who has never been in this situation could never understand.'[19]

Many others just said they were grateful to have their contribution acknowledged for once. But also, predictably, there was a backlash from parents and families, some arguing against the tenet of the speech, which they thought did not acknowledge the contribution of parenting or the benefits of education to society as a whole. The most interesting features both of the political positioning and of the comments were just how extreme and (for the most part) how articulate they were. It was very clear that the majority of the child-free and childless, even if they were prepared to subsidize the children of others, had hitherto felt unacknowledged and ignored.

Ageing and Loneliness

Organizations have now sprung up to try to highlight the difficulties, improve the situation or at least help the childless and child-free deal with the problems they face. Ageing Without Children, AWOC, is a registered community-interest company that aims to highlight and find solutions to the problems for people who are elderly and childless.

How we care for elderly people without offspring is a recognized problem. In 2013 Dr Linda Pickard from London School of Economics warned that: 'A growing family-care gap means that the number of older people in need of care is predicted to outstrip the number of family members able to provide it for the first time in 2017. By 2032, 1.1 million older people in England will need care from their families – an increase of 60 per cent – but the number of people able to care for older parents will have increased by only 20 per cent, creating a shortfall in our collective capacity to care for older generations.'[20]

AWOC's 2015 report on the issues affecting childless people in later life identified six key themes, through focus groups, interviews and life stories.[21] They were:

Invisibility
Being Judged
Who will tell my story?

Being a carer is a trigger point
Practical Support
Disconnect from other generations

The report recommended solutions around the following themes:

A national strategy
Investment in advocacy and intergenerational projects
Better access to advice to help plan for later life
More education and social awareness

From a purely personal perspective, I have my own fears of ageing without having a son or daughter. I think of how we try to support my mum. In more than five decades I have only missed one Christmas with her, and that because I was working in the Middle East and didn't have a holiday. We speak every day, many times a day. Without a child, if I should outlive my husband, what would my contact with the outside world be? Will there be my friends, or will many of them similarly be elderly and infirm and unable to get out and about as much as they may wish to? Who will be my advocate if I can no longer represent myself? But then, I know people with two and three children whose sons and daughters rarely visit, who make a duty phone call once a week, once a month, or for birthdays and holidays. It's not something that can be solved by childbirth; it's not something particular to those who do or do not have a family. Rather it's about the loneliness of our society – a lack of caring, a selfish inward-looking perspective that runs through so much of our way of living. Selfishness,

despite popular opinion, is not the sole preserve of those
without children.

The assumption remains that care in later life, and everything that entails, will fall to your children. Robin Hadley
from AWOC summarizes the issue like this: 'Public services,
especially social care and the NHS generally, assume that
there are adult children around to help fill the gaps in
services. So, for example, that there is probably an adult child
around to run someone to appointments, help with tasks like
cleaning and shopping, remind people to take medication,
help with exercises, change dressings, etc. The system is not
geared up for people without family to help them and at the
same time reductions in public spending mean that many
services that were there to help fill this gap now longer exist.
Consequently people ageing without children can be left
without support and help at a time when they need it most.'[22]

Government pronouncements substantiate this assumption. In early 2017 David Mowat MP, then Undersecretary
of State for Care and Support –the so-called Care Minister
– suggested that people have as much responsibility to care
for their own parents as they do to care for their children.
It's a rather idealistic stance, even disregarding the fact that
having children is a choice, whereas having parents is an
inevitability. For example, it ignores the housing difficulties
in much of the country, where couples living in a studio flat
within commuting distance of their work just wouldn't have
the room or be able to afford to take in an elderly parent, no
matter how much they might wish to.

The government abnegation of responsibility goes beyond
Mowat. The former Families Minister, Tim Loughton,
conjured up a vision of generations of Mediterranean

families living closely together, supporting each other, caring for each other.[23] He neglected to mention those that don't have any family around them. I am reminded of our three years in Italy, a country I love, where I nevertheless felt more excluded from society by being childless and in my forties than I have in any other. Although the society in our small coastal town was centred on parenting, much of Italy is choosing to forgo having a family. The International Centre for Family Studies (CISF) in Milan reported in 2010 that over half of all couples in Italy are childless and that 19.5 per cent of people they interviewed were reluctant to have children for economic reasons. Others cited the size of their flats and houses and the impossibility of finding anything bigger.[24] The choice of childlessness is viewed as a national problem by Francesco Belletti, the director of CISF. He sees the choice as the result of limited facilities and support for people who might otherwise have chosen to become parents. While he commends some local moves to encourage families through sympathetic planning and financial support, he argues that: 'The role of family associations and no profit organizations should be strengthened in planning policies, in providing services, in evaluating outputs, in every level of public administration. Some good examples can be reported at local level (i.e. in Trentino, or in Castelnuovo del Garda), but a long way is still ahead, to build in Italy a family friendly and participated welfare.'[25]

The Mediterranean is not the only region where an unrealistic image of family life exists in the minds of British ministers. In 2013, three years before Loughton's pronouncement, the then Health secretary, Jeremy Hunt, had expressed similar views. We should, he suggested, be more like Asian countries and take in our elderly relatives. Leaving aside the obvious question as to what happens if you don't have children to look after you, some of the most ostracized and victimized childless people I met were in Asia. It is also, almost exclusively, women who do the caring. In Sri Lanka, for example, according to an academic study, 90 per cent of the care-givers identified and interviewed were female, with respondents saying 'daughters made better care-givers because of the "natural instinct" of mothering, and the stronger loyalty women felt towards their parents.'[26] So much for any hope of equality.

In a newspaper opinion piece, Hans Schattle, professor of political science at Yonsei University in Seoul, South Korea, cites reports of old age homes 'plagued by filthy conditions including the stench of excrement and body odour' and observes that 'nearly half the population over sixty-five lives in poverty and the suicide rate among the elderly has more than doubled in the past decade.'[27]

In other parts of Asia, people are increasingly opting for a child-free, often single, lifestyle. Entitled 'post-familialism', the preference for smaller families is seen as the result of a move away from more traditional religious values to secular ones, as well as women's increased autonomy and rejection of 'sharply defined maternal roles'.[28] Japan has the most rapidly declining rate of birth: 'By 2010, a third of Japanese women entering their thirties were single, as were roughly one in five of those entering their forties – that is roughly eight times the percentage in 1960, and twice as many as in 2000. By 2030, according to sociologist Mika Toyota, almost one in three Japanese males may be unmarried by age fifty'.[29]

A report by Age UK observed that Japan is trying to support

the change to much less reliance on informal family care for elderly relatives by launching long-term universal healthcare insurance. But it's clear that the true ramifications of demographic transformation will need a far bigger overhaul of the support offered to older people internationally.

With loneliness being one of the most cited issues facing the elderly childless, any government strategy should include networks and systems to try to alleviate it. The Jo Cox Commission on Loneliness was established following the murder of the Labour MP Jo Cox in 2016, and is a cross-party think tank involving numerous high-profile organizations such as Age UK, the British Red Cross and the Royal Voluntary Service. It aims to propose positive steps we can take to combat loneliness in our society. The slogan #happytochat is used to involve people in the wider community, to encourage them to seek out older people and start up a conversation. However, their report on loneliness and ageing was based on the views of respondents from Gransnet, so did not deal with the specific nature of the isolation that may be suffered by those who don't have family.

By developing their own online community AWOC have provided an alternative social point for those who do not want to have friendly conversations about children and grandchildren, because in some instances, especially for those who were unable to have their own family, such topics can be painful as well as unfulfilling. 'I felt excluded because I wasn't a mum, and now I feel excluded because I don't have grandchildren.'[30]

'Ageing Without Children sounds just what I am looking for! I disagree with many of the former comments, and wonder if they are from people with children and grandchildren? Of course it's not all you talk about, but it is a central subject and those of us with no family (older or younger, or estranged) feel very, very lonely when we have nothing to contribute on the subject of children.'[31]

Until governments internationally recognize the needs of a minority that is steadily increasing and address the key issues of elderly advocacy, care and loneliness, without presuming that there will be family members prepared to pick up the burden, the situation cannot improve. In many countries, the childless and child-free will continue to pay more tax, work longer hours for more years, receive fewer benefits in their lifetime, leave a smaller carbon footprint on the planet and financially support others in their choice to have and raise a family, but receive no extra, much-needed support when they are advanced in years with nobody to turn to. Their punishment for not having children is to be ignored by the state that they have contributed so much to.

A Short Note on Doubt and Politics

In July 2016 there is a furore in the media in the UK. Andrea Leadsom is in competition with Theresa May for the leadership of the Conservative Party after David Cameron resigns, following the country's vote to leave the EU. In support of her own campaign, Leadsom uses the fact that she has children, unlike May, who has previously spoken of her regret that she and her husband cannot. My Twitter feed cascades with indignation that motherhood and the ability to be prime minister should be thus conjoined. Some positions are not much better than Leadsom's, though, such as one beginning, 'I have nephews/nieces etc. and I'm sure May does too, they will give her a stake in the future.' The world has gone mad, albeit briefly, and when I look at other feeds, outwith the safety of my friends and followers, I find a general consensus: many, many people believe we only really care about people we are biologically related to (and thus will somehow take greater care for 'our' future if we have descendants of our own). I also find outright misogyny – which kind of childless woman are you? Up-for-it sex addict? Or kindly maiden aunt? Single and frustrated? Too ugly for your husband?

Despite my arguing and the ridiculous content of some of the tweeting, in the midst of it all I begin to unravel. What I had thought was all behind me returns to haunt my wakefulness, because once again my childlessness makes me sleepless. I've been reconciled for more than ten years to the fact that I will not have a child. But the fact remains that I have never felt what it is like to have something grow inside me. I am untethered by something that is illogical, even cruel, and I am lessened in my own eyes. I doubt everyone. I hear people with children saying, Of course you don't need to be a parent to care about the future; but simultaneously I fight down uncertainty of my own which says, Yes, it is different for me, it must be, because a part of you will inhabit this putative, imaginary future, and a part of me will not. I rail against it silently. I do not have to be biologically related to someone to care that they have a future – of course I don't; the assertion is absurd, but yet, but yet.

I think of friends, colleagues, my editor, my agent, my neighbour, the father of my goddaughter, my husband, and I wonder if in some part of their mind they judge me too, but suppress their own feelings, because they are kind, because they know it is not of my own choosing. Do they ever think – silent, unshared thoughts, fleeting ideas they try to supress in themselves – 'She's not a mother, she doesn't understand', or, 'If she was a mother, she would be better at that, or kinder, or more caring, or just different in a better way.' For a time, I have no confidence that this is not so, and I cannot help it. But then I am calm again. My husband logically says he is not a father either, and is in fact irritated by the whole notion – of course, people may think that, but so what? I envy him the 'so what'. Perhaps because in my secret, dark heart of doubts I am afraid somehow that they are right, that my logic has failed. I have no way of knowing.

A Short Note on Presumption

In the United States men have more negative perceptions of the child-free than women, although they are less likely to be stigmatized if they themselves choose not to become parents.[1]

But what of the childless – is it better to be an object of pity than of unkind presumptions?

I don't know the answer. I do know that I got very tired at one point of people saying how sorry for me they were, how awful it must be. Most studies differentiate clearly between women who are infertile and the way they are perceived and those who are child-free, yet it seems an odd thing to measure, because in the real world who actually knows the reason why you are childless beyond your immediate circle and those rude enough or thoughtless enough to ask?

Most people are curious. I speak from experience. From years of being asked outright, or having to suffer gentle hints as to when there might be the 'patter of little feet'. My identity is inextricably linked to my recalcitrant womb. And while statistically men may view someone without children more negatively, may see the female role as that of mother, it's the women who puzzle me most.

I don't disagree that all women should get behind better working conditions for mothers, but I don't understand why mothers don't then get behind blatant discrimination against the childless in matters such as inheritance tax or EITC or politics.

Even in my highly supportive, very liberal and caring university environment the topic of working mothers (and fathers) frequently arises at union meetings, yet I can't remember an instance when the childless or child-free even merited a mention.

When the baying crowds of social media descended on a child-free woman for having the temerity to propose 'meternity' and then two child-bearing women sat down to mock her on TV, I thought of the chasm between them. Pointedly it was the child-free woman who was accused of letting down the sisterhood – that notional, ideological entity that supposedly groups us together. I couldn't help but wonder if being childless had already somehow excluded her and, if not, where were all the mothers fighting for equality for the childless?

8

Residual Sadness: The Homecoming

The residual sadness still affects us both in waves. I am an only child, so the legacy of my parent's long and happy marriage ends here, with me. I had never really been interested in genealogy in the way that so many of my contemporaries are, in part, I think, because I knew my family stories were so sad, telling of poverty, early deaths. Even my grandmother was sold into service – the unacknowledged slavery of the twentieth century, whereby poor adolescents in their early teens, whose families could not afford to keep them, were offered to wealthy homes as servants in exchange for a sum that might help keep the family that remained at home fed and warm.

Yet infertility gave me more curiosity. In looking back at my ancestry on websites, I find that as recently as two genera-tions ago the women were illiterate; they signed official papers with a cross, their mark. On my father's side there are blacksmiths stretching back as far as I can go, and I think of my lifelong love of horses, the horseshoe that has travelled with me from new home to new home and even now hangs above our door, prongs up so that the luck doesn't run out.

For all the harshness and brevity of their lives, the women of the direct line that stretched back thousands and thousands of years, to the beginning of my family, had all accomplished something that I could not. I have no sisters or brothers. It ends with me.

And so all of this – the thin, unbroken thread of history, the narrative of my parents and of me – is final. I have no real legacy to leave a child in terms of wealth, but some days I think about cascading red hair, a horse rider, a child who loves books, or who can sing and dance, like my mother still does even at her late age. Sometimes I think I see her – an unborn girl, with ginger curls, turning and skipping, restless gracefulness, just out of reach somehow, our never daughter, the one my husband and I could not make together and never will.

It is a pointless day dream. My father's heart beat arhythmically. As I write this we learn that my mum's heart misses one beat in every five. I wonder what mine does. If I had a child, I wonder if he or she would have had this irregular drumming to live their life by.

My husband loved my father, loves my mother, as if they were his own. He too is saddened by the end of things, the end of days, the finite finishing of my family with us. And yet there are many things we have done and seen and been to each other that we might not have done, had there been the presence of a child. There is also the irrefutable fact, reinforced in the course of writing this book, that to be thus is one thing, but to be safely thus is in fact a gift of fortune, because so much worse is possible and prevalent.

On a trip to Loch Awe and Oban, more than a decade after we had come to terms with our state, Alan and I found ourselves in the grey swirling sea mists of December, looking across from Oban Bay to Kerrera and Lismore. It had been a short break brimful of nostalgia – there was the church where we married all those years ago, St Conan, so close to the edge of Loch Awe that you can hear the water from its gardens. There were thoughts of two friends, wedding guests, both lost to us far too soon, and of my dad, whose ashes we had scattered across different parts of this expanse of constantly changing, addictive land, which he had loved, as I now do.

We had had such hope then, in that newly married future, which we had thought began so well, with the simplest of blessings, fair weather and the surprise arrival of my husband's oldest and dearest friend, all the way from Florida, who stood at the altar waiting for our rehearsal to begin. Implicit was always the idea that we would have children and bring them to this place that we thought of as ours. Yet here we were, on a drabber day, at the close of a year, at a much later stage in our lives, knowing that we would not have anyone to bring, to show, to say, 'Look at this, this piece of shingle beach is where your dad proposed to me with two plastic glasses and a bottle of cava.' We would never share the delight of the surprise of it, or the joy, or the way we had always, always agreed that, of course, there would be children, and then there was you.

We look over to the islands and I watch a tethered boat rocking as the wind picks up. I recall the little independently run boats that used to run from Oban to Mull when I was in my teens and twenties, and how I loved the small daughter of the captain of one of those tourist boats, would cradle her and sing to her when her father brought her on those short sails to the castle across the water. I wonder what became of her. She will be all grown up now. Would I have been fertile in my teens, I wonder, my very early twenties? By my mid-twenties, I know most probably I was not. But I did not know my husband then, and to conceive of these years and years without him in them, but with a child by someone else, is as unfathomable to me as the ocean that turns the colour of the landscape here before me – grey on slate on granite, with white, white foam.

I am resigned, then, no more than that; happy still, in spite of it, for the simple pleasure that my husband and I share in being here. I write to one of my oldest and dearest friends of our middle-aged sentimentality, and hope he will tell his daughter, my godchild, that our wedding was a lovely day for him too, as his was for us.

I am reminded of Charles Lamb's essay *Dream Children: A Reverie*. Lamb was a childless bachelor, his life devoted to caring for his sister, and in this essay he imagines two fictitious children. The daughter is reminiscent of an unrequited love whose name was Alice. Both children are saddened by the story of the death of Lamb's brother, but their faces begin to fade 'till nothing at last but two mournful features were seen in the uttermost distance'. The faded faces speak to him more loudly than voices, remind him, 'We are not of Alice, nor of thee, nor are we children at all.' His realization that they 'are nothing; less than nothing, and dreams' comes as he awakes, a bachelor in an armchair, his sister by his side.

For me, here is what remains after the faces of the never-born have gone. The inexorable changes that come in ebbs and flows, the hours and minutes when my lack of progeny means that I must somehow do, achieve, become more than what I am, because there will be nothing left afterwards. My parents' happy marriage and all the myriad, countless bequests to me – from red hair to impatience, cleverness, passion and the acts of simple good manners – end with me. Yet, with time, there are also moments of quiet relief. By finding joy in the life that I have, I am freed from the prison of 'what if', and realize that this moment, this time, is precious too, and would not have happened if it had all come out differently. I have a beloved Dutch goddaughter, and a Chinese godson, named after my father. These small mercies, quiet pleasures, honours bestowed, are all such precious offerings that I can no longer wish that things had been different.

Sadly, of course, it cannot be like this for all of the women I have met. Even if they find consolation in friendship or love, the strictures of a society that has condemned them to silence and belief in their own failure prevail. But perhaps if their voices are heard, it can change, and even if they can never have the children that they long for or lost or that were taken from them, they can one day still find some peace in what remains. I hope it can be so.

Notes

Introduction

1 See Mandelbaum, D. G. (1974) *Human Fertility in India: Social Components and Policy Perspectives*, University of California Press
2 Beckett, S. (1984) *Collected Shorter Plays of Samuel Beckett*, Faber and Faber, p. 241

Those Who Long

1 See Naseef Nassar (1985) 'Wad 'al-mar'ah fi ah al-Dasatir al-Arabiyah', *al-waddah* 1:9, quoted in Y. Haddad and John Esposito (ed.) (1997) *Islam, Gender and Social Change*, p. 6
2 See https://www.alarabiya.net/articles/2010/11/08/125311.html
3 Hadith cited as *sahih* (authentic) by Shaykh Al-Albaani in *Irwa' al-Ghaleel*, 1784
4 http://www.who.int/reproductivehealth/topics/infertility/multiple-definitions/en/
5 Fido, A. (2004) 'Emotional Distress in Infertile Women in Kuwait', *International Journal of Fertility and Women's Medicine*, 49:1, 24–8
6 Abolfotouh et al. (2013) 'Knowledge, Attitude, and Practices of Infertility Among Saudi Couples', *International Journal of General Medicine*, 6, 571
7 Ibid., 563–73

8 'Surah Ash-Shura', *The Quran*, 42:49–50

9 See, for example, Robert Fisk, 'Scarred by the Savage Lash of Islamic Justice', *Independent*, 12 October 1995

10 According to Abū Hurayra, the Prophet said *al-ʿayn uḥakk un*, 'The evil eye is a reality' (al-Bukhārī, commentary of al-Kasṭallānī on the *Ṣaḥīḥ*, viii, 390, 463). See P. Bearman et al. (eds) (2005) *Encyclopaedia of Islam*, second edition, Brill

11 See Vijayakumar, Lakshmi (2015) 'Suicide in Women', *Indian Journal of Psychiatry*, 57:6, 233–8

12 Unisa, Sayeed (1999) 'Childlessness in Andhra Pradesh, India: Treatment Seeking and Consequences', *Reproductive Health Matters*, 7:13, 62

13 Ibid.

14 Mehta, Bhamini, and S. Kapadia (2008) 'Experiences of Childlessness in an Indian Context: A Gender Perspective', *Indian Journal of Gender Studies*, 15:3, 44–441

15 Vijayakumar, 'Suicide in Women', 233–8

16 Accounts taken from the Indo-Asian News Service, 15 February 2011; *The Telegraph*, Calcutta, 19 January 2012; *The Times of India*, 14 March 2014; *TNN*, 19 November 2015

17 Names and details of locations have been changed to preserve anonymity

18 See http://www.starsfoundation.org.uk/awards/organizations /reach-india; accessed 19 June 2017

19 Kordvani, A. H. (2002) 'Hegemonic Masculinity, Domination and Violence Against Women', paper presented at University of Sydney, http://www.austdvclearinghouse.unsw.edu.au/con ference per cent20papers/Exp-horiz/Kordvani.pdf; accessed 19 June 2015

20 See, for example, Sabale, Kowli, et al. (2012) 'Working Conditions and Health Hazards in Beedi Rollers Residing in the Urban Slums of Mumbai', *Indian Journal of Occupational and Environmental Medicine*, 16:2, 72–4

21 Ireland, M. (1993) *Reconceiving Women: Separating Motherhood from Female Identity*, Guilford Press, p. 18

22 See Pearce, Tola Olu (1999) 'She Will Not be Listened to in Public: Perceptions Among the Yoruba of Infertility and Childlessness in Women', *Reproductive Health Matters*, 7:3

23 Ibid., 74

24 'Jo', personal communication, May 2016

25 Melanie Notkin, 'The Truth About the Childless Life', *Huffington Post*, 1 August 2013, http://www.huffingtonpost.com/melanie-notkin/the-truth-about-the-childless-life_b_3691069.html; accessed 16 May 2017

26 Bibi Lynch, 'Mothers, Stop Moaning!', *Guardian*, 31 March 2012

27 Bibi Lynch, 'Do Not Brand Me a Failure', *Guardian*, 29 October 2016

A Short Note about Love

1 Frost, Robert (1916) 'Hyla Brook', *Mountain Interval*, Henry Holt

Those Who Believe

1 All superstitions to do with falling pregnant; the last was one we used to say when I was at school: sitting on a wall would give you a chill and you wouldn't be able to have a baby when you were grown up

2 See Ferris, Father Daniel (1878) *The Life of St Mary Frances of the Five Wounds of Christ*, M. H. Gill

3 See http://www.panagiatinou.gr/eng/; accessed 19 May 2016

4 https://www.pregnancybyfaith.com/

5 This quote is from Rev. Fr Dr Christopher Flesoras, but there are many others. See https://www.goarch.org/-/infertility-and-the-intercessions-of-saints-joachim-anna; accessed 29 June 2017

6 This story is based on a *Christian Science Monitor* article of 3 December 2003, 'Deadly Rites Spark Indian Action: Authorities Fight Tantrism, Linked to 25 Killings This Year', as well as a conversation through an interpreter with a villager

who requested anonymity. Some slight details differ from those in the *Washington Post* piece of 29 November 2003. In such cases I have followed the facts as presented in the interview.

7   The account of the witches' camps in Ghana is largely taken from Yaba Badoe's excellent work on the region: Badoe, Y. (2011) 'The Witches of Gambaga: What it Means to be a Witch in the Northern Region of Ghana', *Jenda: A Journal of Culture and African Women's Studies*, 19; it is also informed by her moving documentary film *The Witches of Gambaga*

8   See Tabong, Philip Teg-Nefaah, and Philip Baba Adongo (2013) 'Understanding the Social Meaning of Infertility and Childbearing: A Qualitative Study of the Perception of Childbearing and Childlessness in Northern Ghana', *PLoS ONE*, 8:1

9   Ibid., 6

10   http://www.fertilityfairness.co.uk/wp-content/uploads/2015/11/FFPoliticalBriefing2015.pdf; last accessed 19 October 2016

11   All details of IVF provision taken from ibid.

12   Melanie asked not only that I change her identity but also that I not specify her region because she is seeking legal advice about the ramifications of her story

13   Kjaer, T., et al. (2014) 'Divorce or End of Cohabitation Among Danish Women Evaluated for Fertility Problems', *Acta Obstetricia et Gynecologica Scandinavica*, 93, 269–76

14   Robert Winston, 'Why I'm Ashamed of Exploitation in the IVF Industry', *Daily Mail*, 4 May 2017

15   Ibid.

16   Ibid.

17   Ibid.

18   Sher Fertility, *I Believe*, https://www.youtube.com/watch?v=b10OQ0qPT9A; accessed 30 June 2017

19   Rogers, C. (1951) *Client-Centered Therapy: Its Current Practice, Implications and Theory*, Constable

20   See Nina Chohan, 'Infertility "Still a Taboo Subject",

Survey Suggests', http://www.bionews.org.uk/page_357538. asp; accessed 3 July 2017

A Short Note on the Naming of Things

1 Nahar, Papreen, and S. van der Geest (2014) 'How Women in Bangladesh Confront the Stigma of Childlessness', *Medical Anthropology Quarterly*, 28:3, 388

2 Pujari, Sucharita, and S. Unisa (2014) 'Failing Fatherhood: A Study of Childless Men in Rural Andhra Pradesh', *Sociological Bulletin*, 63, 23

3 Tabong, P., and P. Adongo (2013) 'Infertility and Childlessness: A Qualitative Study of the Experiences of Infertile Couples in Northern Ghana', *BMC Pregnancy and Childbirth*, 13:72

Those Who Were Denied

1 'Nordic Eugenics: Here of all Places', *Economist*, 31 August–5 Sept. 1997, pp. 36–7; 'Eugenic Scandal Rocks Scandinavia', *Guardian Weekly*, 31 August 1997, p. 1; for details of the Alberta cases, see D. C. Park and J. Radford (1998) 'From the Case Files: Reconstructing a History of Involuntary Sterilization', *Disability and Society*, 13:3, 317–42

2 Park and Radford, 323

3 Ibid., 326

4 Ibid., 327

5 Ibid., 330

6 Ibid., 332

7 Leilani Muir's own recollection in the documentary *The Sterilization of Leilani Muir*

8 Kalanithi, Paul (2016) *When Breath Becomes Air*, Random House

9 Gibb, L. (1995) *Marimei* Taboos of Kelderash Romanies, *Lore and Language*, 13:1, 73–6

10 Okely, J. (1983) *The Traveller-Gypsies*, Cambridge University Press; Okely has an account of related taboos among English Roma

11 Personal communication, June 1991

12 Names and all identifying features have been altered at her request; the interview was conducted some years ago and at the time Rosa gave me her permission to use it whenever I wished so long as she was not identifiable

13 Personal communication, August 1991

14 See 'Sterilized Roma accuse Czechs', *BBC News*, 12 March 2007, http://news.bbc.co.uk/1/hi/world/europe/6409699.stm

15 *The Sterilization of Roma Women* (2003), Journeyman Pictures

16 Bukovska, Barbara (2003) *Body and Soul: Forced Sterilization and Other Assaults on Roma Reproductive Freedom in Slovakia*, Center for Reproductive Rights and Poradna pre obcianske a l'udské práva

17 See, for example, Naomi Kinsella, 'Case Notes, *I.G. and Others v. Slovakia* [2012] ECHR 1910', 13 November 2012, http://hrlc.org.au/forced-sterilization-of-roma-women-is-inhuman-and-degrading-but-not-discriminatory/

18 The Quipu Project: https://interactive.quipu-project.com/#/en/quipu/intro

19 'Peru's Forcibly Sterilized Women Find Their Voice', *Guardian*, 4 January 2016, https://www.theguardian.com/global-development/2016/jan/04/peru-forced-sterilization-quipu-project-alberto-fujimori; accessed 1 February 2017

20 *Secret Sterilization* (1999), Journeyman Pictures

21 https://interactive.quipu-project.com/#/en/quipu/intro

22 World Health Organization, *Fact Sheet on Female Genital Mutilation*, February 2017, http://www.who.int/mediacentre/factsheets/fs241/en/

23 Almroth, Lars, et al. (2005) 'Primary Infertility After Genital Mutilation in Girlhood in Sudan: A Case-Control Study', *The Lancet*, 366, 385–91

24 The interview with Almroth was in 'Female Genital Mutilation Can Cause Infertility', *New Scientist*, 29 July 2005

25 Ibid.

26 Mwanri, Lillian, and G. J. Gatwiri (2017) 'Injured Bodies,

Damaged Lives: Experiences and Narratives of Kenyan Women with Obstetric Fistula and Female Genital Mutilation/Cutting', *Reproductive Health*, 14:38

27 Ibid., 7–8
28 Ibid.
29 Ibid.
30 Ibid., 10
31 The discussion of China's one-child policy and infanticide is based on Jimmerson, J. (1990) 'Female Infanticide in China: An Examination of Cultural and Legal Norms', *Pacific Basin Law Journal*, 8:1, UCLA School of Law, https://escholarship.org/uc/item/80n7k798; and Croll, E. (ed.) (1985) *China's One-Child Family Policy*, Macmillan
32 Jimmerson, 'Female Infanticide in China'
33 The accounts that follow are taken from Zhang, Weiguo (2007) 'Marginalization of Childless Elderly Men and Welfare Provision: A Study in a North China Village', *Journal of Contemporary China*, 16:51, 275–93. I am grateful to Professor Zhang too for his correspondence and helpfulness. The setting and descriptive details are from my own research and are representative of the region and setting.
34 See, for example, Zhang, Zhenmei, and Mark Hayward (2001) 'Childlessness and the Psychological Well-Being of Older Persons', *Journal of Gerontology*, Series B, 56:5, S311–S32; Dykstra, P., and G. Hagestad (2007) 'Roads Less Taken: Developing a Nuanced View of Older Adults Without Children', *Journal of Family Issues*, 28, 1275–310; Vikström, et al. (2011) 'The Influences of Childlessness on the Psychological Well-Being and Social Network of the Oldest Old', *BMC Geriatrics*, 11:78; Zhang, Weiguo, and Guiping Liu (2007) 'Childlessness, Psychological Well-Being, and Life Satisfaction Among the Elderly in China', *Journal of Cross-Cultural Gerontology*, 22:2, 185–203; Chou, Kee-Lee, and Iris Chi (2004) 'Childlessness and Psychological Well-Being in Chinese Older Adults', *International Journal of Geriatric Psychiatry*, 19:5, 449–57

35 See, for example, Overymer, Daniel, and Lizhu Fan (2006) *Collection of Folk Customs in Handan Area*, Tianjin Chinese Classic Press, pp. 65–6

36 Chen, Houqiang (2006) *Overview of Chen Clan in Cangnan County*, Hangzhou Press; *Cangnan Xian Chen Xing Tong Lan* (2006), Hangzhou Chuban She, 157, discusses the Chen family, who have been in Chenjiabao village since 1250 CE and completed an impressive temple for ancestral worship in 2004, which represents not only their wealth but the fecundity and thus the continuity of their line

A Short Note on Things That Matter

1 See Fairchilds, Cissie C. (2007) *Women in Early Modern Europe 1500–1700*, Pearson Education, p. 87

2 See, for example, Kettering, Sharon (2014) *French Society 1589–1715*, Routledge

Those Who Adapt

1 Nanar, Papreen, and S. van der Geest (2014) 'How Women in Bangladesh Confront the Stigma of Childlessness: Agency, Resilience and Resistance', *Medical Anthropology Quarterly*, 28:23, 381

2 Ibid., 382, but see also Nahar, Papreen, and A. Richters (2011) 'Suffering of Childless Women in Bangladesh', *Anthropology and Medicine*, 18, 327–38

3 Papreen and van der Geest, 'How Women in Bangladesh Confront the Stigma of Childlessness', 383

4 Ibid., 393

5 Ibid.

6 Ibid., 387

7 Todorova, I., and Tatyana Kotzeva (2003) 'Social Discourses, Women's Resistive Voices: Facing Involuntary Childlessness in Bulgaria', *Women's Studies International Forum*, 26:2, 139–51

8 Ibid., 150

9 Hollos, M., and Whitehouse, B. (2008), 'Fertility and the Modern Female Life Course in Two Southern Nigerian Communities', *Ethnology*, 47:1, 23

10 See Njanji, Sue (1998) 'Our Own Gift', *New Internationalist*, 303, in Humanities International Complete Database, and also https://www.globalgiving.org/pfil/688/projdoc.pdf; accessed 7 June 2017

11 See https://www.globalgiving.org/pfil/688/projdoc.pdf p. 2

12 See https://www.changemakers.com/ashoka-fellows/entries/chipo-chedu; accessed 7 June 2017

13 Jangara, Tarisai (2013) 'Female Infertility: Stigma and Heartache', http://www.thezimbabwean.co/2013/02/female-infertility-stigma-and-heartache/; accessed 7 June 2017

14 See http://fertilitynetworkuk.org/wp-content/uploads/2016/06/FACTSHEET-Childless-Coping-Strategies-Toolkit.pdf; accessed 7 June 2017

15 For more details on the *burrnesha*, the *Kanun* and its effect on women's lives, see Mustafa, Mentor, and A. Young, 'Feud Narratives: Contemporary Deployments of *Kanun* in Shala Valley, Northern Albania', *Anthropological Notebooks*, 14:2, 87–107, and 'Last of the *Burrnesha*: Balkan Women Who Pledged Celibacy to Live as Men', *Guardian*, 5 August 2014

16 Keqi's story is taken from Dan Bilefsky, 'Sworn to Virginity and Living as Men in Albania', *New York Times*, 23 June 2008

17 Ibid.

18 Ibid.

19 Ibid.

20 Ibid.

21 Ibid.

22 *Saut Al-Umma* (Egypt), 3 February 2002, as cited in *Al-Quds Al-Arabi* (London), 4 February 2002

23 See https://budourhassan.wordpress.com/2013/05/27/palestinian-women-trapped-between-occupation-and-patriarchy/; accessed 9 June 2017

24 See http://www.al-monitor.com/pulse/originals/2016/09/israel-murder-of-women-in-arab-society-by-contract-ki.html; accessed 9 June 2017

25 See *The Times of Israel*, 18 May 2017, http://www.timesofisrael.com/as-so-called-honor-killers-get-away-with-murder-palestinians-say-law-judges-outdated/

26 Tzoreff, Mira (2006) 'The Palestinian Shahida: National Patriotism, Islamic Feminism or Social Crisis', Yoram Schweitzer (ed.) *Female Suicide Bombers: Dying for Equality*, Jaffee Center for Strategic Studies, Tel Aviv University, p. 20

27 Ibid., p. 14

28 Aysheh's message to Israel, cited in Sjoberg, Laura, and C. E. Gentry (2013) *Mothers, Monsters, Whores: Women's Violence in Global Politics*, Zed Books

29 Schweitzer, Y. (2006) 'Palestinian Female Suicide Bombers: Reality vs Myth', Schweitzer, *Female Suicide Bombers*, p. 20

30 From *Al-Akhbar* newspaper, quoted in Tzoreff, 'The Palestinian Shahida', p. 20

31 From *Al-Akhbar* newspaper, quoted in Issachov, A. (2006) 'The Palestinian and Israeli Media on Female Suicide Terrorists', Schweitzer, *Female Suicide Bombers*, p. 47

32 Ibid. p. 48

33 Silva Mangalika, quoted in Cutter, A. (1998) 'Tamil Tigresses, Hindu Martyrs', *Journal of International Affairs*, Columbia University, http://www.columbia.edu/cu/sipa/PUBS/SLANT/SPRING98/article5.html

34 Menake's story and quotes are taken from Jan Goodwin, 'When the Suicide Bomber is a Woman', *Marie Claire*, 16 January 2008

35 Ibid., p. 12

36 Alhassan, Abbas, et al. (2014) 'A Survey on Depression Among Infertile Women in Ghana', *Bio Med Central*, 14–42

37 See http://www.judiciary.go.ke/portal/assets/filemanager_uploads/Speeches per cent202016/Sitati per cent20J. per cent20-per cent20Woman-Woman per cent20Marriage.pdf; accessed 10 June 2017

38 Kjerland, Kirsten Alsaker (1997) 'When African Women take Wives', *Poverty and Prosperity*, Nordic Africa Institute Occasional Papers No. 6, 2

39 Ibid., 1

40 Njambi, W. N., and A. O'Brien (2000) 'Revisiting "Woman-Woman Marriage": Notes on Gikuyu Women', *National Women's Studies Association Journal*, 12, 1

41 *The Free Lance–Star*, Fredericksburg, Virginia, 29 January 1983

42 Taken from an account in Njambi, 'Revisiting "Woman-Woman Marriage"' 9–10

43 Ibid., 10

44 Ibid., 12

45 Ibid.

46 Ibid.

47 Ibid.

Those Who are Childless Parents

1 Talbot, K. (1998–9) 'Mothers Now Childless: Personal Transformations After the Death of an Only Child', *Omega*, 38, 167–86

2 This was the case for Fiona and Ian Murray, interviewed by Laura Donnelly, *Telegraph*, 14 August 2017, http://www.telegraph.co.uk/women/mother-tongue/9469008/Stillbirth-causes-a-grief-that-hurts-unlike-any-other.html

3 Ibid.

4 O'Leary, Joann, and J. Warland (2013) 'Untold Stories of Infant Loss: The Importance of Contact with the Baby for Bereaved Parents', *Journal of Family Nursing*, 19:3, 324–47

5 http://www.telegraph.co.uk/women/mother-tongue/9469008/Stillbirth-causes-a-grief-that-hurts-unlike-any-other.html

6 Personal communication by Skype, 19 August 2017; all names and locations have been changed in accordance with the interviewees' wishes

7 'Silence After a Stillbirth Is Deafening – and Painful, Say

Parents', *ABC News*, 11 December 2003, http://abcnews. go.com/Health/silence-stillbirth-deafening-painful-parents/ story?id=21166037

8 Barak, Adi, and R. D. Leichtentritt (2014) 'Configurations of Time in Bereaved Parents' Narratives', *Qualitative Health Research*, 24:8, 1090–101

9 Ibid., 1095

10 Ibid., 1096

11 Ibid., 1098

12 Personal communication by Skype, February 2016 – all names have been changed

13 Personal communication by Skype, March 2016 – all names have been changed

14 See Talbot, K. (1996–7) 'Mothers Now Childless: Survival After the Death of an Only Child', *Omega*, 34, 177–89, and Talbot, 'Mothers Now Childless: Personal Transformations'

15 Talbot, 'Mothers Now Childless: Personal Transformations', 167

16 The quotes that follow are from our meeting in February 2017 and from the PeaceWomen website, http://www.peacewomen. org/assets/file/SecurityCouncilMonitor/ArriaFormula/ October2010/biography_visakadharmadasa.pdf

17 Mellibovsky, M. (1996), *Circle of Love Over Death*, Curbstone Books, p. 27

18 Ibid., p. 185

19 Greif, G. (2012) 'The Impact of Child Abduction in Families', *Psychology Today*, https://www.psychologytoday.com/blog/ buddy-system/201205/the-impact-child-abduction-families

20 Boss, P. (1999) *Ambiguous Loss: Learning to Live with Unresolved Grief*, Harvard University

21 Sessions, Hilary R. (2011) *Where's My Tiffany*, iUniverse, p. 302

22 See Tanith Carey, 'Can an Age-Processed Picture of a Dead Child Really Help Bereaved Parents?', *Guardian*, 16 May 2014, https://www.theguardian.com/lifeandstyle/2014/may/16/ age-progressed-picture-dead-child-help-parents

23 National Inquiry into the Separation of Aboriginal and Torres

Strait Islander Children from Their Families (1997) *Bringing Them Home*, evidence 260 by Professor Colin Tatz, Centre for Comparative Genocide Studies, https://www.humanrights. gov.au/publications/bringing-them-home-chapter–1

24 Ibid., p. 9

25 Ibid., submission 186, part III, pp. 30–31

26 Ibid., confidential evidence 143, Victoria

27 https://www.australia.gov.au/about-australia/our-country/ our-people/apology-to-australias-indigenous-peoples; accessed 6 June 2017

28 John Pilger, 'Another Stolen Generation: How Australia Still Wrecks Aboriginal Families', *Guardian*, 21 March 2014

29 Laura Wradjiri, Skype interview, 9 June 2017

30 Ibid.

31 Douglas, H., and T. Walsh (2013) 'Continuing the Stolen Generations: Child Protection Interventions and Indigenous People', *International Journal of Children's Rights*, 21, 59–87

32 Ibid., 60

33 Ibid., 76

34 Ibid., 81

35 Ibid., 82, quoting one of the interviewed lawyers

36 See https://www.tcf.org.uk/

37 See https://www.tcf.org.uk/content/resources/L05-Childless-parents-C12-R1607.pdf

38 Joanna Moorhead, 'They Call Us Childless Parents', *Guardian*, 6 June 2009, https://www.theguardian.com/lifeandstyle/2009/ jun/06/child-bereavement

A Short Note on Kahlo

1 *Querido Doctorcito: The Correspondence of Frida Kahlo and Dr Eloesser* (2007), El Equilibrista, p. 59

2 *The Diary of Frida Kahlo* (1995) Abrams, p. 212

3 Cited by Javier Espinoza, *Guardian*, 12 August 2007, https:// www.theguardian.com/world/2007/aug/12/artnews.art

Those Who Choose: Child-free

1 Pashigan, Melissa (2002) 'Conceiving the Happy Family', *Infertility Around the Globe*, University of California Press, pp. 134–51

2 Morrell, Carolyn M. (1994) *Unwomanly Conduct: The Challenges of Intentional Childlessness*, Routledge

3 See Blackstone A., and M. Stewart (2012) 'Choosing to be a Parent', *Sociology Compass*, 1–10, for a comprehensive account

4 Waren, W., and H. Pals (2013) 'Comparing Characteristics of Voluntarily Childless Men and Women', *Journal of Population Research*, 30:2, 151–70

5 http://www.childlessbychoiceproject.com/the-survey.html; accessed 25 May 2017

6 Cited in Blackstone and Stewart, 'Choosing to be a Parent', 1–10

7 Avison, M., and A. Furnham (2015) 'Personality and Voluntary Childlessness', *Journal of Population Research*, 32, 48

8 Blackstone, A., and M. Stewart (2016) 'There's More Thinking to Decide: How the Childfree Decide Not to Parent', *The Family Journal*, 24:3, 296–303

9 See ibid. and Copur, Zeynep, and Tanya Koropeckyj-Cox (2010) 'University Students' Perception of Childless Parents and Couples in Ankara, Turkey', *Journal of Family Issues*, 31, 1481–506; Koropeckyj-Cox, Tanya, and Gretchen Pendell (2007) 'Attitudes About Childlessness in the United States: Correlates of Positive, Neutral and Negative Responses', *Journal of Family Issues*, 28, 1054–82

10 *RT News*, 11 August 2014, https://www.rt.com/news 20179588-iran-bans-permanent-contraception/; accessed 31 May 2017

11 However, in 2017 an Iranian official called for the sterilization of homeless women – he said 'they reproduce like hatching machines and as their children have no guardians, they sell them'; see *The New Arab*, 1 January 2017, https://www.alaraby.

co.uk/english/News/2017/1/1/Iran-official-says-homeless-women-should-be-sterilized

12 Callan, Victor J. (1985) 'Perceptions of Parents, the Voluntarily and Involuntarily Childless: A Multidimensional Scaling Analysis', *Journal of Marriage and the Family*, 47, 1045–50

13 Polit, Denize F. (1978) 'Stereotypes Relating to Family-Size Status', *Journal of Marriage and the Family*, 40, 105–14

14 See, for example, Dever, M., and L. Saugeres (2004) 'I Forgot to Have Children! Untangling Links Between Feminism, Careers and Voluntary Childlessness', *Journal of the Association for Research on Mothering*, 6:2, 116–26; Letherby, G., and C. Williams (1999) 'Non-motherhood: Ambivalent Autobiographies', *Feminist Studies*, 25:3, 719–28; Koropeckyj-Cox, T., et al. (2007) 'Through the Lenses of Gender, Race, and Class: Students' Perceptions of Childless/Childfree Individuals and Couples', *Sex Roles*, 56, 415–28

15 Vidad, Felizon C. (2009) *Mental Health Professionals' Perceptions of Voluntarily Childless Couples*, PhD thesis, Antioch University, USA

16 Professor Eric Heinze, personal communication

17 Antony Heaven, personal communication

18 National Centre for Health Statistics, https://www.cdc.gov/nchs/fastats/contraceptive.htm; accessed 31 May 2017

19 See, for example, http://www.independent.co.uk/news/uk/home-news/woman-who-never-wanted-children-wins-nhs-sterilization-battle-a7030481.html; accessed 30 May 2017

20 See Bartz, D., and J. A. Greenberg (2008) 'Sterilization in the United States', *Reviews in Obstetrics and Gynecology*, 1:1, 23

21 Bartz and Greenberg, 'Sterilization in the United States', 23–32

22 Ibid., and also Catherine Pearson, 'Meet the 20-Somethings Who Want to be Sterilized', *Huffington Post*, 24 October 2014, updated 28 October 2014

23 Who should pay for that choice is a separate issue and will be dealt with later in the section

24 Benn, Piers, and Martin Lupton (2005) 'Sterilization of Young,

Competent and Childless Adults', *British Medical Journal*, 4 June, 330:7503, 1323–5

25 Seeley, Bri, 'What it Really Feels Like to be a Child-Free Woman', *Huffington Post*, 16 August 2014, updated 16 October 2014

26 http://www.nhs.uk/Conditions/contraception-guide/Pages/vasectomy-male-sterilization.aspx;   http://www.nhs.uk/conditions/contraception-guide/pages/female-sterilization.aspx; accessed 27 May 2017

27 http://blog.practicalethics.ox.ac.uk/2015/05/legally-competent-but-too-young-to-choose-to-be-sterilized/; accessed 27 May 2017

28 Katherine Bindley, 'NYPD to Women of Brooklyn's Park Slope: Don't Wear Shorts or Dresses', *Huffington Post*, 30 November 2011, http://www.huffingtonpost.com/2011/09/30/nypd-to-women-of-south-park-dont-wear-shorts-or-dresses_n_989539.html; accessed 28 May 2017

29 Wolfendale, Jessica (2016) 'Provocative Dress and Sexual Responsibility', *Georgetown Journal of Gender and the Law*, 17:1

30 Pugh, Jonny, 'Legally Competent, But Too Young to Choose to Be Sterilized?', *Practical Ethics*, 7 May 2015, http://blog.practicalethics.ox.ac.uk/2015/05/legally-competent-but-too-young-to-choose-to-be-sterilized/#more-11179

31 Seeley, 'What it Really Feels Like to be a Child-Free Woman'

32 Lisa Hymas, personal communication

33 Anna Williams, personal communication

34 http://oregonstate.edu/ua/ncs/archives/2009/jul/family-planning-major-environmental-emphasis; accessed 30 May 2017

35 Hymas, Lisa, 'I Decided Not to Have Children for Environmental Reasons', *Guardian*, 29 September 2011

36 Stephanie Kirchgaessner,'Pope Francis: Not Having Children is Selfish', *Guardian*, 11 February 2015

37 A pseudonym

38 Malthus, T. (1798) *An Essay on the Principle of Population*, J. Johnson

39 https://www.populationmatters.org/the-issue/overview/; accessed 7 March 2017

40 Skype interview with Lisa Hymas, 10 June 2017

41 Basten, Stuart (2009) 'Mass Media and Reproductive Behaviours: Serial Narratives, Soap Opera and Telenovelas', *The Future of Human Reproduction*, University of Oxford Working Paper 7

42 Ibid.

43 Ibid., 6

44 World Population Review for Mexico, http://worldpopulationreview.com/countries/mexico-population/; accessed 12 June 2017

45 Chatterji, S., 'Looking Back at *Hum Log*', *India Together*, 25 July 2008, http://www.indiatogether.org/humlog-women--2

46 Rieder, Travis, and Rebecca Kukla, 'As Environmental Catastrophe Looms, is it Ethical to Have Children?', *Foreign Policy*, 31 May 2017

47 https://carmelitesistersocd.com/2014/spiritual-mother hood/; accessed 9 March 2017

48 Ibid.

49 Sister Brittany, personal communication; you can follow Sister Brittany on Twitter as @sisterb24

50 Ibid.

51 Ibid.

52 https://carmelitesistersocd.com/2014/spiritual-mother hood/, and also Congregatio pro Clericis, 8 December 2007, http://www.clerus.org/clerus/dati/2008-01/25-13/Adoration.pdf

53 See Ireland, *Reconceiving Women*, p. 111

54 Mary, personal communication

55 Hauswirth, Frieda (1932) *Purdah: Status of Indian Women*, Vanguard Press

56 Blackstone and Stewart, 'There's More Thinking to Decide'

57 *Chicago Tribune*, 22 July 2015, http://www.chicagotribune.com/lifestyles/sc-fam-0728-childless-by-chance--20150721-

story.html; accessed 1 June 2017

58 Morrell, *Unwomanly Conduct*
59 Vicky Smith (a pseudonym), personal communication
60 Inhorn, Marcia, and Frank Van Balen (2002) *Infertility Around the Globe*, University of California Press, p. 5
61 Goffman, Erving (1963) *Stigma: Notes on the Management of Spoiled Identity*, Prentice-Hall, quoted in Park, Kristin (2002) 'Stigma Management Among the Voluntarily Childless', *Sociological Perspectives*, 45:1, 21–45
62 Park, 'Stigma Management', 36–37

A Short Note on Femininity and Womanhood

1 She also includes the works of Jean Genêt
2 Nin, Anais (1992) *Incest*, Penguin, pp. 380, 381
3 Bair, D. (1995) *Anais Nin: A Biography*, Bloomsbury
4 See Sady Doyle, 'Before Lena Dunham, there was Anaïs Nin', *Guardian*, 7 April 2015, https://www.theguardian.com/culture/2015/apr/07/anais-nin-author-social-media
5 See Jarczok, A. (2017) *Writing an Icon: Celebrity Culture and the Invention of Anais Nin*, Swallow Press

A Short Note on the Voices of History

1 'Kahun Medical Papyrus' or 'Gynaecological Papyrus' (translation by Stephen Quirke), Petrie Museum of Egyptian Archaeology, UC 32057, pp. 1–2
2 Radice, Betty (trans.) (1963) *The Letters of the Younger Pliny*, Pliny to Calpurnia, Book 7, Letter 5, Penguin; https://erenow.com/biographies/the-letters-of-the-younger-pliny/9.html

Punished for Being Without Children in the West

1 See Shapiro, G. (2014) 'Voluntary Childlessness: A Critical Review of the Literature', *Studies in the Maternal*, 6:1

2 Gillespie, R. (2000) 'When No Means No: Disbelief, Disregard and Deviance as Discourses of Voluntary Childlessness', *Women's Studies International Forum*, 23: 2, 223–34

3 See Shapiro, 'Voluntary Childlessness', 10

4 Bays, Annalucia (2017) 'Perceptions, Emotions and Behaviours Towards Women Based on Parental Status', *Sex Roles*, 76, 138

5 See https://www.gov.uk/government/publications/inheritance-tax-main-residence-nil-rate-band-and-the-existing-nil-rate-band/inheritance-tax-main-residence-nil-rate-band-and-the-existing-nil-rate-band; accessed 21 July 2017

6 McDonnell, Kelly, 'New Inheritance Tax Rules Discriminate Against the Childless', *Wills and Probate News*, 26 August 2015

7 'End Inheritance Tax (IHT) Discrimination Against the Childless', https://petition.parliament.uk/petitions/105736

8 Holzer, H. (2015) 'Should the Earned Income Tax Credit Rise for Childless Adults?', *IZA World of Labor*, https://wol.iza.org/articles/should-earned-income-tax-credit-rise-for-childless-adults/long

9 Marr, C. and B. DaSilva (2016) 'Childless Adults Are Lone Group Taxed Into Poverty', *Center on Budget Policy Priorities*, https://www.cbpp.org/research/federal-tax/childless-adults-are-lone-group-taxed-into-poverty; accessed 21 July 2017

10 Carroll, Laura, 'The Brutal Truth About Being Childless at Work', *Fortune*, 7 November 2015, http://fortune.com/2015/11/07/truth-about-childless-at-work/; accessed 2 June 2017; see also Notkin, Melanie (2014) *Otherhood: Modern Women Finding a New Kind of Happiness*, Penguin

11 Amy Blackstone quoted in Carroll, 'The Truth About Being Childless'

12 Ibid.

13 Davies, Anna, 'I Want All the Perks of Maternity Leave – Without Having Any Kids', *New York Post*, 28 April 2016

14 Betts, Hannah, 'Childless Women Should Get Maternity Too', *Telegraph*, 2 May 2016

15 See Chalmers Chartered Accountants, https://www. chalmershb.co.uk/news/business-news/archive/article/2016/ April/tuc-study-finds-significant-wage-gap-between-working-fathers-and-childless-men; *Metro*, 25 April 2016, http:// metro.co.uk/2016/04/25/men-with-children-earn-more-than-those-without–5838317/; http://www.bbc.co.uk/news/business–36126584

16 Allardyce, Jason, 'Nicola Sturgeon: The Baby I Lost', *Sunday Times*, 4 September 2016

17 Meotti, Giulio, 'Europe's Childless Leaders Sleepwalking Us to Disaster', 6 May 2017, https://www.gatestoneinstitute. org/10306/childless-europe; accessed 2 June 2017

18 *Aljazeera*, 16 June 2016, http://www.aljazeera.com/news/2016/ 06/turkey-erdogan-childless-women-incomplete–160606 042442710.html; accessed 5 June 2017

19 https://www.youtube.com/watch?v=9RBj57fOSVM; accessed 2 June 2017

20 Pickard, L. (2013) 'A Growing Care Gap? The Supply of Unpaid Care for Older People by Their Adult Children in England to 2032', *Ageing and Society*, http://eprints.lse. ac.uk/51955/

21 https://ageingwithoutchildren.files.wordpress.com/2015/05/ awocsurvey15.pdf

22 http://www.robinhadley.co.uk/more/ageing-without-children-awoc.shtml

23 Swinford, Steven, 'Parents Responsible for Care of Their Elderly Mothers and Fathers as Much as Their Own Children, Minister Says', *Telegraph*, 31 January 2017

24 White, Hilary, 'Over Half of Italian Families Childless: Report', 24 March 2010, https://www.lifesitenews.com/news/ over-half-of-italian-families-childless-report; accessed 5 June 2017

25 A full account of Belletti and his team's recommendations can be downloaded from http://www.ohchr.org/documents

26 Watt, Melissa, et al. (2014) 'Care-giving Expectations and

Challenges Among Elders and Their Adult Children in Southern Sri Lanka', *Ageing and Society*, 34:5, 838–58

27 Schattle, Hans, 'Asia is a Terrible Model for Elderly Care, Jeremy Hunt', *Guardian*, 18 October 2013; https://www. theguardian.com/commentisfree/2013/oct/18/jeremy-hunt-elderly-care-asia

28 Kotkin, Joel (2012) 'The Rise of Post-Familialism: Humanity's Future', *New Geography*, http://www.newgeography.com/ content/003133-the-rise-post-familialism-humanitys-future; accessed 5 June 2017

29 Kotkin,   'The   Rise   of   Post-Familialism', http://www.newgeography.com/files/The%20Rise%20 of%20Post-Familialism%20(ISBN9789810738976).pdf, 3

30 AWOC, 'Loneliness: It's Not Enough to be Happy to Chat, You Have to be Ready to Listen Too', https://awoc. org/2017/03/29/loneliness-its-not-enough-to-be-happy-to-chat-you-have-to-be-ready-to-listen-too/

31 Comment on Gransnet by Vicmee, 11 July 2017

A Short Note on Presumption

1 Koropeckyj-Cox, T. and G. Pendell (2007) 'The Gender Gap in Attitudes About Childlessness in the United States', *Journal of Marriage and Family*, 69: 4

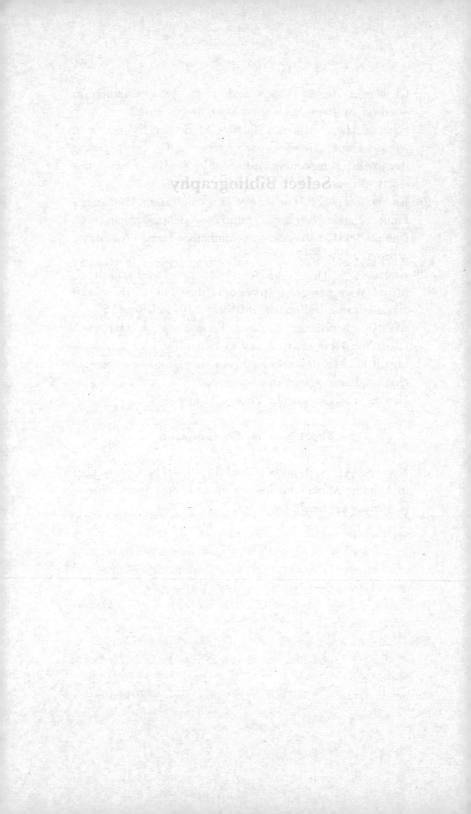

Select Bibliography

Abolfotouh et al. (2013) 'Knowledge, Attitude, and Practices of Infertility Among Saudi Couples', *International Journal of General Medicine*, 6, 563–73

Alhassan, Abbas, et al. (2014) 'A Survey on Depression Among Infertile Women in Ghana', *Bio Med Central*, 14–42

Almroth, Lars, et al. (2005) 'Primary Infertility after Genital Mutilation in Girlhood in Sudan: A Case-Control Study', *The Lancet*, 366, 385–91

Badoe, Y. (2011) 'The Witches of Gambaga: What it Means to be a Witch in the Northern Region of Ghana', *Jenda: A Journal of Culture and African Women's Studies*, 19

Barak, Adi, and R. D. Leichtentritt (2014) 'Configurations of Time in Bereaved Parents' Narratives', *Qualitative Health Research*, 24:8, 1090–110

Bartz, D., and J. A. Greenberg (2008) 'Sterilization in the United States', *Reviews in Obstetrics and Gynecology*, 1:1, 23–32

Basten, Stuart (2009) 'Mass Media and Reproductive Behaviours: Serial Narratives, Soap Opera and Telenovelas', *The Future of Human Reproduction*, Oxford University Working Paper 7

Blackstone, A., and M. Stewart (2012) 'Choosing to be a Parent', *Sociology Compass*, 1–10

Blackstone, A., and M. Stewart (2016) 'There's More Thinking to Decide: How the Child-free Decide Not to Parent', *The Family Journal*, 24:3

Bukovska, Barbara (2003) *Body and Soul: Forced Sterilization and*

Other Assaults on Roma Reproductive Freedom in Slovakia, Center for Reproductive Rights and Poradna pre obcianske a l'udské práva

Callan, Victor J. (1985) 'Perceptions of Parents, the Voluntarily and Involuntarily Childless: A Multidimensional Scaling Analysis', *Journal of Marriage and the Family*, 47, 1045–50

Chou, Kee-Lee, and Iris Chi (2004) 'Childlessness and Psychological Well-Being in Chinese Older Adults', *International Journal of Geriatric Psychiatry*, 19:5, 449–57

Copur, Zeynep, and Tanya Koropeckyj-Cox (2010) 'University Students' Perception of Childless Parents and Couples in Ankara, Turkey', *Journal of Family Issues*, 31, 1481–506

Croll, E. (ed.) (1985) *China's One-Child Family Policy*, Macmillan

Daum, Meghan (2015) *Selfish, Shallow and Self-Absorbed*, Picador

Day, Jodi (2013) *Living the Life Unexpected*, Bluebird: London

Dever, M., and L. Saugeres (2004) 'I Forgot to Have Children! Untangling Links Between Feminism, Careers and Voluntary Childlessness', *Journal of the Association for Research on Mothering*, 6:2, 116–26

Douglas, H., and T. Walsh (2013) 'Continuing the Stolen Generations: Child Protection Interventions and Indigenous People', *International Journal of Children's Rights*, 21, 59–87

Dykstra, P., and G. Hagestad (2007) 'Roads Less Taken: Developing a Nuanced View of Older Adults Without Children', *Journal of Family Issues*, 28, 1275–310

Fido, A. (2004) 'Emotional Distress in Infertile Women in Kuwait', *International Journal of Fertility and Women's Medicine*, 49:1, 24–28

Fisk, Robert, 'Scarred by the Savage Lash of Islamic Justice', *Independent*, 12 October 1995

Gayle, Claudine, and J. Rymer (2016) 'Female Genital Mutilation and Pregnancy: Associated Risks', *British Journal of Nursing*, 25:17

Gibb, L. (1995) '*Marimei* taboos of Kelderash Romanies', *Lore and Language*, 13:1, 73–6

Goffman, Erving (1963) *Stigma: Notes on the Management of Spoiled Identity*, Prentice-Hall

Haddad, Y., and John Esposito (ed.) (1997) *Islam, Gender and Social Change*, Meridian

Hollos, M., and B. Whitehouse (2008) 'Fertility and the Modern Female Life Course in Two Southern Nigerian Comunities', *Ethnology*, 47:1, 23

Inhorn, Marcia, and Frank Van Balen (2002) *Infertility Around the Globe*, University of California Press

Ireland, M. (1993) *Reconceiving Women: Separating Motherhood from Female Identity*, Guildford Press

Issachov, A. (2006) 'The Palestinian and Israeli Media on Female Suicide Terrorists', Yoram Schweitzer (ed.) *Female Suicide Bombers: Dying for Equality*, Jaffee Center for Strategic Studies, Tel Aviv University

Jimmerson, J. (1990) 'Female Infanticide in China: An Examination of Cultural and Legal Norms', *Pacific Basin Law Journal*, 8:1, UCLA School of Law

Lisle, Laurie (1996) *Without Child*, Ballantine Books

Kahlo, Frida (1995) *The Diary of Frida Kahlo*, Abrams

Kjaer, T., et al. (2014) 'Divorce or End of Cohabitation Among Danish Women Evaluated for Fertility Problems', *Acta Obstetricia et Gynecologica Scandinavica*, 93, 269–76

Kjerland, Kirsten Alsaker (1997) 'When African Women take Wives', *Poverty and Prosperity*, Nordic Africa Institute Occasional Papers No. 6

Kordvani, A. H. (2002) 'Hegemonic Masculinity, Domination and Violence Against Women', paper presented at University of Sydney, http://www.austdvclearinghouse.unsw.edu.au/conference per cent20papers/Exp-horiz/Kordvani.pdf

Koropeckyj-Cox, Tanya, and Gretchen Pendell (2007) 'Attitudes About Childlessness in the United States: Correlates of Positive, Neutral and Negative Responses', *Journal of Family Issues*, 28, 1054–82

Koropeckyj-Cox, Tanya, et al. (2007) 'Through the Lenses of Gender, Race, and Class: Students' Perceptions of Childless/Childfree Individuals and Couples', *Sex Roles*, 56, 415–28

Lavania, Vinita (2006) *Social Consequences of Sterility and Infertility*, Rawat Publications

Letherby, G., and C. Williams (1999) 'Non-Motherhood: Ambivalent Autobiographies', *Feminist Studies*, 25:3, 719–28

Marsh, M., and W. Ronner (1996) *The Empty Cradle*, Johns Hopkins University Press

May, Elaine Tyler (1995) *Barren in the Promised Land*, Basic Books

Mehta, Bhamini, and S. Kapadia (2008) 'Experiences of Childlessness in an Indian Context: A Gender Perspective', *Indian Journal of Gender Studies*, 15:3, 44–441

Morrell, Carolyn M. (1994) *Unwomanly Conduct: The Challenges of Intentional Childlessness*, Routledge

Mwanri, Lillian, and G. J. Gatwiri (2017) 'Injured Bodies, Damaged Lives: Experiences and Narratives of Kenyan Women with Obstetric Fistula and Female Genital Mutilation/Cutting', *Reproductive Health*, 14:38

Nahar, Papreen, and S. van der Geest (2014) 'How Women in Bangladesh Confront the Stigma of Childlessness: Agency, Resilience and Resistance', *Medical Anthropology Quarterly*, 28:23, 381

Nahar, Papreen, and A. Richters (2011) 'Suffering of Childless Women in Bangladesh', *Anthropology and Medicine*, 18, 327–38

Nin, Anaïs (1993) *Incest*, Penguin

Njambi, W. N., and A. O'Brien (2000) 'Revisiting "Woman-Woman Marriage": Notes on Gikuyu Women', *National Women's Studies Association Journal*, 12:1

Notkin, Melanie (2014) *Otherhood: Modern Women Finding a New Kind of Happiness*, Seal Press

Okely, J. (1983) *The Traveller-Gypsies*, Cambridge University Press

Overymer, Daniel, and Lizhu Fan (2006) *Collection of Folk Customs in Handan Area*, Tianjin Chinese Classic Press

Park, D. C., and J. Radford (1998) 'From the Case Files: Reconstructing a History of Involuntary Sterilization', *Disability and Society*, 13:3, 317–42

Park, Kristin (2002) 'Stigma Management Among the Voluntarily Childless', *Sociological Perspectives*, 45:1, 21–45

Pashigan, Melissa (2002) 'Conceiving the Happy Family', *Infertility Around the Globe*, University of California Press

Pearce, Tola Olu (1999) 'She Will Not be Listened to in Public. Perceptions Among the Yoruba of Infertility and Childlessness in Women', *Reproductive Health Matters*, 7:13

Polit, Denise F. (1978) 'Stereotypes Relating to Family-Size Status', *Journal of Marriage and the Family*, 40, 105–14

Rosof, B. D. (1994) *The Worst Loss: How Families Heal from the Death of a Child*, Henry Holt

Sabale, Kowli, et al. (2012) 'Working Conditions and Health Hazards in Beedi Rollers Residing in the Urban Slums of Mumbai', *Indian Journal of Occupational and Environmental Medicine*, 16:2, 72–4

Schweitzer, Y. (2006) 'Palestinian Female Suicide Bombers: Reality vs Myth', Yoram Schweitzer (ed.), *Female Suicide Bombers: Dying for Equality*, Jaffee Center for Strategic Studies, Tel Aviv University

Sjoberg, Laura, and C. E. Gentry (2013) *Mothers, Monsters, Whores: Women's Violence in Global Politics*, Zed Books

Tabong, Philip Teg-Nefaah, and Philip Baba Adongo (2013) 'Understanding the Social Meaning of Infertility and Childbearing: A Qualitative Study of the Perception of Childbearing and Childlessness in Northern Ghana', *PLoS ONE*, 8:1

Talbot, K. (1996–7) 'Mothers Now Childless: Survival After the Death of an Only Child', *Omega*, 34, 177–89

Talbot, K. (1998–9) 'Mothers Now Childless: Personal Transformations After the Death of an Only Child', *Omega*, 38, 167–86

Todorova, I., and Tatyana Kotzeva (2003) 'Social Discourses, Women's Resistive Voices: Facing Involuntary Childlessness in Bulgaria', *Women's Studies International Forum*, 26:2, 139–51

Tzoreff, Mira (2006) 'The Palestinian Shahida: National Patriotism, Islamic Feminism or Social Crisis', Yoram Schweitzer (ed.) *Female Suicide Bombers: Dying for Equality*, Jaffee Center for Strategic Studies, Tel Aviv University

Unisa, Sayeed (1999) 'Childlessness in Andhra Pradesh, India: Treatment Seeking and Consequences', *Reproductive Health Matters*, 7:13, 62

Victor, Barbara (2004) *Army of Roses*, Constable and Robinson

Vidad, Felizon C. (2009) 'Mental Health Professionals', Perceptions of Voluntarily Childless Couples', PhD thesis, Antioch University, USA

Vijayakumar, Lakshmi (2015) 'Suicide in Women', *Indian Journal of Psychiatry*, 57:6, 233–8

Vikström, et al. (2011) 'The Influences of Childlessness on the Psychological Well-Being and Social Network of the Oldest Old', *BMC Geriatrics*, 11:78

Waren, W., and H. Pals (2013) 'Comparing Characteristics of Voluntarily Childless Men and Women', *Journal of Population Research*, 30:2, 151–70

Zhang, Weiguo (2007) 'Marginalization of Childless Elderly Men and Welfare Provision: A Study in a North China Village', *Journal of Contemporary China*, 16:51, 275–93

Zhang, Weiguo, and Guiping Liu (2007) 'Childlessness, Psychological Well-Being, and Life Satisfaction Among the Elderly in China', *Journal of Cross-Cultural Gerontology*, 22:2, 185–203

Zhang, Zhenmei, and Mark D. Hayward (2001) 'Childlessness and the Psychological Well-Being of Older Persons', *Journal of Gerontology*, Series B, 56:5, S311–S32

Films

The Sterilization of Roma Women (2003) Journeyman Pictures
Lunik IX: A Short Documentary (2012) Artur Conka

Acknowledgements

Above all I offer my heartfelt gratitude to the many, many men and women from across the globe who replied to my calls and requests to share their stories.

Thanks also to Susan Davies, Gill Hartley, Abi May, Jules Radford, Michael Mbito, Professor Weiguo Zhang, Professor Catherine Reissler, Lesley Pyne, Meresa Atieno, Aba Mbuto, Catherine Hill, Kate Brien and Jodie Day, Tony Hetherington and Debbie Stuart, Dr Vivienne Francis, Andrew Gallacher, Martha Stuart, Giovanna Cecchi, Laura Lyons from Grandmothers Against Removals, Rawat Publications, Ageing Without Children, the Quipu Project and Dr Sylvia Shaw for directing me to them.

The film-maker and writer Yaba Badoe very generously shared her transcripts with me. I hope she feels I have put them to good use. Thank you. In Sri Lanka Visaka Dharmadasa welcomed me to her home. Dr Chamil Rathnayake helped make my trip both trouble-free and enjoyable, and Priyan Wijerathne of the Kandalama Hotel went well beyond what I might have expected in helping me understand more of Gunurathne's story. Bri Seeley, Sister Brittany and Lisa Hymas all shared their thoughts with me at length. Priyanka Banerjee, Partha Pratim Rudra and

Abhinaba Majumdar from Reach India gave me access to stories that would otherwise have been unheard.

Antony Heaven, Professor Eric Heinze, Professor Gregory Dart and Helen Logan all made helpful suggestions.

Some of the travel to research this book was made possible by a sabbatical from Middlesex University. I am very lucky to have a small group of colleagues and former students that I also think of as friends, as well as support from the wider department. Thank you especially for facts, linguistic peculiarities, contacts and kindnesses: Dr Alejandro Abraham-Hamanoiel, Dr Helen Bendon, Yasmin Alibhai-Brown, Dr Maggie Butt, Dr Anna Charalambidou, James Charlton, Professor Billy Clark, Professor Paul Cobley, David Cottis, Margaret Davis, Sophia Kostoglou-Drakopoulou, Louise Huggett, Anna Kujawska, Dr Magnus Moar, Nayomi Roshini, Dr Frank Shennan, Dr Catherine Ann Cullen and Carole-Anne Upton.

Kelly Da Silva's Dovecote community offers a very special, safe, free online space for women who are struggling with childlessness.

A generous grant from the Society of Authors enabled me to travel to Sri Lanka and conduct interviews there. Their financial support of writers is unparalleled.

My editor at Granta, Max Porter, has provided a great deal of cheerfulness and his usual remarkable talent to help make this book what it is. Natalie Shaw, Ka Bradley and Christine Lo all worked the usual Granta magic and Daphne Tagg was a careful and sympathetic copy editor. I still feel extraordinarily fortunate to have my amazing agent, Peter Straus at RCW.

My dear, dear friend Dr Michael Newton read and commented on early drafts, as well as making me the godmother of his lovely Hannah. Professor Paul Komesaroff has been a tireless and inspirational example of how much good one person can do in the world. Charles Palliser and Carl Rollyson have been as kindly supportive as they always are to fellow writers. My former Doha students Kinda Murad and Aisha Althani still give me friendship and gifts more than a decade after I taught them. Both are wonderful mothers who have been sympathetic and understanding of the sadness of childlessness. Alessia Bianciardi befriended me when I was isolated in a foreign country and just learning to come to terms with our new future.

Thanks also to Robin Fairfield, who offered lovely dinners and ballet outings as an escape from my computer, to Liz Leyshon, who hosted weekends in Somerset, to Diego Lourenco, for visits and lunches and lifts, and to my erstwhile travel companion, Chris Burkinshaw.

As always, writing takes its toll on those we are closest to. My mum, Jessie Gibb, is ceaselessly patient, endlessly kind. Had I become a mother, I would have had an incredible example to follow. This book is for my husband, Alan Wesselson. For all that it has taken me to write it, it seems a tiny, insignificant thing in the face of what he gives to me.